Imagine Doing Better

Imagine Doing Better

Why Policies Backfire and How Prevention Thinking Can Change Everything

Paul J. Fleming

JOHNS HOPKINS UNIVERSITY PRESS

Baltimore

© 2025 Johns Hopkins University Press
All rights reserved. Published 2025
Printed in the United States of America on acid-free paper
9 8 7 6 5 4 3 2 1

Johns Hopkins University Press
2715 North Charles Street
Baltimore, Maryland 21218
www.press.jhu.edu

Library of Congress Cataloging-in-Publication Data is available.

ISBN 978-1-4214-5286-9 (print format)
ISBN 978-1-4214-5287-6 (ebook)

A catalog record for this book is available from the British Library.

*Special discounts are available for bulk purchases of this book.
For more information, please contact Special Sales
at specialsales@jh.edu.*

EU GPSR Authorized Representative
LOGOS EUROPE, 9 rue Nicolas Poussin, 17000, La Rochelle, France
E-mail: Contact@logoseurope.eu

Another world is not only possible, she is on her way. On a quiet day, I can hear her breathing.
—Arundhati Roy

Dedicated to my children and all the future children in the world

Contents

Contents

PART III **Action**

Preface: What Will Our Great-Great-Great-Great-Great Grandchildren Say?

Two hundred years from now, the sun will rise on a world that is hard to imagine. Children will live in that world, waking up to a reality built on the choices we are making today. Those children may not think of us, but I think of them. I wonder what brings them joy. I wonder what they are excited about. I wonder what they feel scared of. I wonder what opportunities they will have. I wonder if they feel safe. I wonder if they are proud or ashamed of the choices their ancestors are making.

We have all been the children that previous generations wondered about. Our ancestors imagined what our lives would be like. George Orwell imagined the year of my birth in *1984*. Octavia Butler's Earthseed series imagined what the decade of the 2020s would be like—30 years before it happened. In both cases, the authors described a dystopian future that charted the potential consequences of the choices being made when they were writing. Their imagination of our future informed and fueled countless readers to build a better future than those Orwell and Butler described.

It can be hard to imagine what life will be like in 200 years. But we have to try, because we still have a chance to shape that future. The society we build today through our actions, policies, and budgets will flow through time to affect that child, their family, their neighbors, and the other people, plants, and animals they share their world with. If we can imagine doing better, it can help orient us to the actions needed in the present day that can build the future we want and need. As Robin D. G. Kelley has written in his groundbreaking book *Freedom Dreams: The Black Radical Imagination*, "the map to a new world is in the imagination."[1]

Sometimes, it can be challenging to imagine doing better. That better future is obscured by the present-day wars, hatred, disinformation, dehumanization, and violence we are living through. It can make it seem as if we are on an unchangeable path toward a dystopian future. But, collectively through our imagination, reflection, and action, we can make a better world possible.

This book describes a future-oriented way to look at the choices we make as a society. I advocate for the use of a prevention mindset to imagine, reflect, and take action to create the transformative change we need. A prevention mindset identifies the root causes of societal problems and focuses society on preventing harms before they happen. Using a future-oriented prevention mindset reinforces an important lens that we can use to reflect on the harms of our current choices and take action to plant the seeds for a better future.

* * *

The Iroquois Nation anointed new chiefs by imploring them to lead and make decisions thinking about their community seven generations into the future.[2] This Native American concept, also used by other Indigenous groups, ensures a long-term perspective when making important decisions for a society.[3] I live and work on land taken from the Anishinaabe people of the Three Fires Confederacy (the Ojibwe, Odawa, and Potawatomi) by the European settlers who formed the new US government.[4] Many government leaders then and now have seemed to disregard the wisdom of this "seven generations" philosophy.

The European settlers instead created a nation with public policies that viewed the land and people as resources that could be used to build wealth. Perhaps they *were* thinking generations ahead. Many of the early policymakers in the United States were able to pass their wealth—the land they took, the people they enslaved, and the natural resources they pulled from the land—on to their descendants which made those descendants wealthy and powerful. That intergenerational wealth passed down across generations shows up in the inequalities that we see today.[5] The idea of prioritizing family wealth instead of community and planetary well-being has entrenched public policies in the United States that cannot carry us another seven generations. We are reaching a breaking point.

If our planet and country are thriving in the year 2225—about seven generations in the future—it will be because we have made transformational changes to our ways of being. The course we are on now has the potential to lead to climate catastrophe, economic collapse, and political ruptures if we do not take action to change direction. In 2225, our descendants seven generations into the future will be opening their eyes for the first time to the world around them. What world will they see? What world will they inherit? That world will be very different from our own, either because of actions taken to transform our policies or because of consequences resulting from a lack of action.

I have three young children. According to life expectancy data, they might live until about the year 2100. By that time, climate projections suggest the global temperatures will be several degrees higher and well past the "point of no return" with severe consequences. In the United States, it is unclear whether the growing political polarization will continue to a point that breaks our country. It is very possible that gun violence, restrictions on reproductive rights, wealth inequality, and racism will get worse in the coming decades.

Or it is possible that strong countervailing forces will swing the pendulum toward collectivism and sustainable communities that promote repair and reconciliation and build toward a better future for all. We are at a turning point, and thinking generations into the future can help us see our current situation from a new perspective and take action to make a better world possible.

Even though I know the path toward catastrophe is a possibility, I actively hold onto hope that we will take the alternative path. Maintaining that hope, and *acting* on it, is part of living and working for future generations.

I am hopeful that we can shift course to a society that abandons exploitative and extractive public policies and instead creates public policies based on principles of equity, collectivism, sustainability, and human dignity. If we can manage to do this, future generations will look at our present day with confusion. What questions will our descendants living in a transformed society in 2225 ask about our life in the 2020s?

If poverty is bad for health and well-being, why would it be legal to pay a worker a poverty wage?

Why spend billions of dollars to keep people locked up when that money could be invested in rehabilitation?

When we knew how harmful pollution and climate change was, why were corporate profits prioritized over the well-being of our home planet?

Why did the myth of "meritocracy" and "equal opportunity" persist when there were such large inequalities in school funding?

Why were police with guns the solution for people in crisis? If preventing harms was the goal, why not spend that money on things that helped people avoid stealing or being violent in the first place?

Why did they allow so many preventable deaths simply because people did not have the money to access health care?

It is a bit of a struggle to understand how we will get to the point where all of our descendants can ask these questions and critique our society without courting debate or controversy. But we have to remind ourselves that we too are descendants of people living seven generations ago.

For many of us, seven generations ago would have been people living during the first few decades that the United States existed. Today, without much controversy, we can condemn the system of chattel slavery because abolitionists organized and fought to transform our society. We can condemn our government's genocide of Native Americans because of the Indigenous Peoples Movement that shone a light on the atrocities committed. We can condemn harsh working conditions early in the industrial revolution because labor organizers took action to show how harmful those practices were. Our country's policies and practices have evolved in the past seven generations because of residents who came together and worked to radically transform our society. We can critique and condemn because some people living at that time used imagination, reflection, and action to radically transform the world.

Some of those evolutions have been positive, but some have also been negative. In recent decades, we have criminalized drugs and become reliant on prisons and policing to solve societal problems and disproportionately targeted those tools at communities of color. We have created a transportation system that is dependent on expensive, inefficient, personal vehicles rather than publicly funded and efficient transportation options. We have created an expensive health care system that often prioritizes profit over community health and can be extremely challenging for some residents to access. More recently, our federal government has backtracked on civil rights and racial equity issues.

These changes have occurred because of policy choices that residents and their elected representatives have made. Choices about where to invest funds, where to give tax breaks, what to regulate, and what to prioritize. Those choices have led us to the conditions we live in today: an incredibly well-resourced society with vast inequities and an unsustainable future. The choices we all make in the coming years—at the ballot box and in our decisions to work collectively for change—will determine the future conditions our great-great-great-great-great grandchildren will live in.

* * *

In this book, I apply a *prevention mindset* to a broad range of issues affecting our society. The prevention mindset is commonly used within public health—the field where I teach, do research, and engage in community projects. This mindset can help us to recognize how our current public policies fall short in getting at the root cause of issues we care about. It can help us identify alternative investments to prevent problems before they occur. Issues of health, safety, climate change, education, and others can be seen in a different light when applying a prevention mindset. I summarize research showing the surprising harms of our public policy choices and tell the story of how we ended up with these outdated policies. I advocate for an alternative vision for our society: one based on principles of prevention and addressing root causes of bad outcomes rather than merely trying to address symptoms after the fact. I hope it can be a resource and guidebook for people who want to use our vast resources to transform our country so that everyone has the opportunity to live and thrive.

In my job as a public health professor, I teach the next generation of people working in public health about a prevention mindset. I teach about "interventions." How do we intervene to change policies, change the environment, and change people's behaviors in order to prevent harms before they happen? My teaching draws on decades of research on this topic and lessons from my own research in collaboration with communities to promote equity, health, and well-being. This book aims to convey some of these same lessons for people who want to make a better future possible. What does the evidence say about the root causes of inequity and harm in our society? And what can we possibly do about it?

* * *

I am someone who has been on the winning end of many of the public policies I describe in this book that disadvantage and harm people who have fewer resources because of who they are and where they grew up. I am often on the winning end because of who I am and the resources that have been available to me throughout my life. I am a white man who grew up in a leafy suburb of Chicago and had the support and resources needed to eventually become a professor of public health at a prestigious university. I now live in a leafy neighborhood of Ann Arbor with my wife and three young children. Daily, I benefit from advantages related to my social class, my race, my gender, my education, my citizenship, and my ability status. Those advantages are baked into our society through the public policy and budgeting choices that we have made over generations. This book is not a memoir of my advantages, although I think it is important to clearly state who I am, and I will continue to offer personal examples throughout the book.

While I benefit from many advantages, it is also critical to point out that our policies still can harm people like me and everyone else in our society. For example, I live down the street from a small lake that has been polluted with chemicals that can cause cancer. It was polluted because of lax oversight of a local

corporation. Weak environmental regulations disproportionately hurt some groups, including poor, Black, or Indigenous
communities, but they ultimately cause harm to us all. Heather
McGhee's *The Sum of Us* explains the legacy of US policies designed to harm Black Americans—policies related to public
parks, the cost of college, and the health care system—and how
they have made everyone in society worse off.[6] The goal cannot
be solely to make sure everyone has the same advantages as me
(although that is a great place to start). Instead, we need to imagine doing better and create policies that will minimize harm
and enable all people to thrive.

I did not always fully appreciate how our public policies could
harm people. It was only when I began working in public health
that I started to better understand the ideas that are contained
in this book. I began to see that the ideas and principles of a prevention mindset used in public health could have a profound
effect if we applied them to issues across our society.

The work that I do in public health focuses on working with
community-based organizations to improve health for the groups
that suffer the worst health outcomes. Over the years, I have
partnered with grassroots groups run by undocumented immigrants, community clinics serving our country's poorest neighborhoods, support groups for people living with HIV, activist
groups trying to reduce police violence, and local government
agencies serving their community. Unsurprisingly, doing this
work across these many different groups, I see the same thing
over and over. The people who have the worst outcomes tend to
be people who have been historically marginalized and disem-
powered by our public policies: people of color, those with low
formal education levels and low income, the disabled, and the
undocumented. This inequity was particularly stark during
the COVID-19 pandemic, when a lot of people like me had no
close family members die or be hospitalized, whereas Black

Americans or poor Americans were much more likely to have people close to them die.[7] The reality is that this same dynamic plays out with most of our health outcomes and other metrics related to education or financial security.

The field of public health holds values of *equity* and *prevention* to be foundational. I write this book from those values. Today, we see vast inequities in our society, many of them caused by public policies and budgetary choices that are causing harm for certain members of society and benefiting others. To increase *equity* in our society, we need to make different choices. And we need to move toward a mindset that *prevents* problems before they happen. Climate catastrophe is one easy example. If we do not try to prevent it, disaster is almost certain. But this mentality can be used for a range of policy issues important to us.

I write from the premise that most of us share similar values of fairness, compassion, honesty, and kindness, even if we might have a million different ideas about what it means to enact those values. I am not naive to think that every reader will agree with me on how to create public policies to live out these values. But I hope that you will approach the book with an open mind and be willing to consider that our current policies and systems may not be the best way to live out these values as a society. The changes that are needed may not be tweaks around the edges but a fundamental reorientation of how we think about our public policies and public budgets. A better world *is* possible. Together, we can imagine doing better, engage in critical reflection, and take action—just like some of our ancestors seven generations ago did. We can make a better world where all of our great-great-great-great-great grandchildren can thrive.

Imagine Doing Better

PART I

Imagination

CHAPTER 1

Possibilities

Don't ask the question, "What do we have now and how can we make it better?" Instead ask, "What can we imagine for ourselves and the world?"

—Mariame Kaba

When my son was six years old, he was just starting to get a grasp of money. He started to understand that things cost money and that we did not have an unlimited supply of it. But it was confusing for him because we almost always paid for things using a credit card. He was six during the height of the pandemic when we often did grocery delivery. Our food would just show up on our doorstep, and he had no idea that money was even exchanged.

So, my son's experience with money was mostly small bits of cash that he might receive as a birthday present or coins he found on the street or in the couch. His aunts know that sending a crisp $10 bill through snail-mail is way more exciting than his dad saying, "Your aunt just sent me a Venmo payment for you!" He started to collect his newfound wealth in a rotund ceramic piggy bank that was a gift from his grandmother.

One time, we were visiting a big-box store that had a small section of toys illuminated in the glow of endless neon lights overhead. The toy section had two short aisles, practically nothing compared to Target or a legitimate toy store. He zeroed in on a plastic toy dinosaur that he begged me to buy him. It was a T. rex, about a foot tall, with nothing particularly notable except that it could make a measly "roar" that was scratchy and muffled at the touch of a button. It cost about $12, and my response to his request was "no."

Given that our house already seemed to be overflowing with toys and that my son wasn't even much of a dinosaur enthusiast, it didn't seem like a wise use of money to me. Even so, I reminded him that *he* could buy it. I reminded him that his aunts sometimes send him money and that he sometimes finds coins that eventually could add up to $12. He would have to budget his limited resources and decide if this toy was worth it.

The thing is, my son became a bit fixated on the idea of *this dinosaur*. He had a one-track mind about it simply because he saw it and remembered it. It was a tangible thing that he had seen and was aware he could buy. So, if he had $12, he would buy *that dinosaur*.

I saw that he was mentally stuck. Anyone who knows a six-year-old knows that they have things they love and are obsessed with. I can tell you that my son was *not* actually obsessed with dinosaurs at that age. He had some interest, but when he was six, he actually was obsessed with soccer, animals, pretending to ninja-chop things, bike riding, and watching TV. Also, "animals" is selling it short: he was obsessed with *predators*—of all types—and made his parents and sisters play predator/prey games. I have had to casually graze the grasslands of our playroom pretending to be an antelope while a "lion" stalks me from behind some toys and then pounces to kill and eat me. I have had to pretend to be a polar bear that is darted by a scientist who then performs examinations. Our playroom transformed regularly from the savanna to the jungle to the arctic and was home to other predator species such as jaguars and cheetahs.

Given his obsession with animals, I couldn't help but wonder: Does he know that there may be other toys out there he might like *even better*? After all, he had grown up as a pandemic kid with a public health professor dad and a nurse for a mom. We had been quite cautious about outings into indoor spaces during the first two years of the pandemic. Rarely did we bring him to stores, and especially toy stores.

In that one store we visited, the toy selection was limited. He saw his options and gravitated to the dinosaur. Wonderful. But before he is going to spend that $12 of his own money on a toy, does he know there are other stores? Does he know that other stores would have an entirely different set of toys? Does he know that he could buy a toy lion? A soccer ball? A set of animal toys? Or even some cheap pet like a goldfish or hermit crab? He was limiting his options to that one store in that one location rather than seeing the plethora of options for his $12. And if he branched out from the "toy" category, that $12 could be spent on food from his favorite local taco joint, a visit to the pool, a puzzle, or any other thing. His budget was limited but the options were really only limited by his imagination. His vision for what was possible was stuck on that one store. And he wanted *that dinosaur*.

He bought that dinosaur. And it provided about 23 minutes of joy. Perhaps 23 minutes of joy for a six-year-old is all that $12 dollars can buy. But, if he could have just expanded his mind and had more imagination, he might have gotten a better outcome. I suspect a toy lion would have gotten more than 23 minutes of play out on the grasslands of our playroom. The joy from that would likely even be spread out over days or weeks, even months!

* * *

Spending $12 without thinking through all your options is usually no big deal. But what about $6 trillion? That was the US federal budget for 2024. How much of that spending and those policy choices were limited by our collective imagination? What if we stepped back from a decision to spend more than $700 billion on the military and instead asked ourselves what the goals are for our money?

If my son's goal was joy, we could have processed all the things that make him feel joy. If our goal as a society is safety, then what are the things that make us feel safe? If our goal is health, what are all the things that contribute to our being healthy? Medicaid and Medicare—our biggest federal health expenditures—certainly are not the only things that help us be healthy. Our health is also about the pollution in the air, our access to safe housing, our ability to receive a high-quality education, and many other things.

When crafting budgets and policies, we often begin by looking at what we have now and how we can make it better. At first, this sounds reasonable. But activist and community organizer Mariame Kaba reminds us that this type of mindset will not lead us to the society that we need. Just like my son's narrow thinking did not help him. Kaba urges us: "Instead ask, 'What can we imagine for ourselves and the world?'"[8]

We all have a tendency to get stuck in status quo thinking. We stay within the same store. Yes, we are going to try and figure out what the best possible purchase is in that store, but we struggle to venture outside it to consider other possibilities. This is similar to the difference between reform and transformation as described by Russell Ackoff. Ackoff notes that reform changes some behaviors but keeps the overall structure in place, whereas transformation changes the structure and the way it functions.[9] He also notes that transformative changes "are radical (go to the roots of the system) or even revolutionary."

Other thinkers imagining what social change should look like—French social theorist André Gorz, for example, or present-day prison abolitionists—have made a similar distinction between "reformist reforms" (those that do not change the existing

structure) versus non-reformist reforms (those that help to transform the system to prioritize human needs).[10,11] Reformist reforms are those policy choices where we limit ourselves only to
the options within one store rather than allow ourselves to consider the full range of possibilities.

Imagination and gaining a new perspective on our society, our
policies, and our budgets can help us break out of this limited
mindset. Ruha Benjamin wrote on the importance of dreaming
different worlds in *Imagination: A Manifesto*. In the book, she
underscores the need for "a collective imagination, as when we
imagine different worlds together, writing shared stories and
plotting futures in which we can all flourish."[12] We need to be
able to envision alternative futures for our communities—futures
that might take a completely different path than the one we are
currently on.

*   *   *

Our imaginations are often limited because we *think* we know
how the world works. But we sometimes cannot see clearly what
is in front of us. The late David Foster Wallace, acclaimed writer
and essayist, illuminates this in a story he told at the beginning
of a graduation speech he gave at Kenyon College in 2005:

> There are these two young fish swimming along and they happen to
> meet an older fish swimming the other way, who nods at them and
> says, "Morning, boys. How's the water?" And the two young fish
> swim on for a bit, and then eventually one of them looks over at the
> other and goes, "What the hell is water?"[13]

When you are in the middle of something, it can be hard to see
what the alternatives are. It can be hard to imagine a world that
looks and feels different from the one you inhabit. It is difficult
know what water is if you don't know what dry land is. Indeed,
what is water? It takes a dedication to imagination, hope, and

sometimes trying to step outside your own world to see things from a new perspective.

NASA's Apollo 8 mission in 1968 was the first spacecraft with a human crew to leave Earth's orbit. The first time humans left our own world and saw things from a new perspective. Its space mission was to orbit the moon in preparation for NASA's planned moon landing the following year. When the astronauts reached the moon and began orbiting, they saw something no one had ever seen before. They saw the Earth rise above the horizon of the moon. Since the dawn of human history, people have observed the moon and the sun rising above Earth's horizons, but the Apollo 8 astronauts were the first to witness an *Earthrise*, a perspective-shifting visual. Astronaut William Anders was quick thinking enough to grab a camera and take a photograph.

The "Earthrise" photograph is one of the most iconic images of the 20th century and one you have likely seen. The vast gray bumpy surface of the moon is up-close and in the foreground. The small-looking Earth is just above the moon's horizon and set against a jet-black sky. The shape of our blue-green marble was lit by the sun in such a way that it matched the shape of the moon in its gibbous phase (somewhere between half and full). The more familiar sight that humans are used to—one with an earthen landscape in the foreground and the moon hovering above the horizon—is completely upended and transformed. The Earthrise image disabuses us from a perspective of our planet that is vast and limitless. The image demands that we see not only the beauty of Earth but also its relative tininess in the vastness of open space. Earth is finite, with clear edges and bounds. Contrast that with nature photographs—or our own lived experience dwelling on Earth—that show endless plains, forests, or oceans, implying the expansiveness and limitlessness of our planet. The Earthrise photo invited us to rethink our perspective.

It is a magnificent image and one I grew up being able to see. But humans living decades before 1968 could only imagine such a perspective, and they may never have taken the opportunity to do so. When the world saw this image for the first time, it was as if those fish in David Foster Wallace's story suddenly had someone share an image of a beach or coastline with them for the first time. The fish probably were too absorbed in what they knew to consider an alternative perspective.

The Earthrise photo is credited with launching the modern environmental movement. Astronaut Anders said, "We came all this way to explore the moon, and the most important thing is that we discovered the Earth." The very first Earth Day was in April 1970, just 15 months after the Earthrise photo was taken. Reflecting on the photo, Kathleen Rogers, president of the Earth Day Network, says: "Earthrise instilled a sense of urgency for those who were already on the front lines battling pollution and making the case that our health and planet were in danger. Earthrise was a confirmation of the righteousness of the endeavor, building confidence in what was a scattered movement into something more cohesive."[14] The new perspective prompted many to make changes to how they lived and the laws and policies they felt were necessary for us to thrive.

* * *

Space travel—or the photography from astronauts and telescopes—is not the only way to step outside our world. Art, literature, and film broaden our perspectives in imagining alternative futures. Consider books or movies that create alternative realities or envision the future. Thought-provoking movies like *The Matrix* let us see our current world from a new and different perspective. Watching Keanu Reeves dodge bullets in slow motion was certainly incredible, but what was really mind-blowing about *The Matrix* was the idea that humans are trapped inside a simulated reality. It prompted audiences to view our relationship with technology differently.

Literature like Octavia Butler's prescient Earthseed series (*The Parable of the Sower* and *The Parable of the Talents*) narrates a story that causes us to question the choices we are making in the present day. Although it was written in the 1990s, it tells the story of the sociopolitical collapse of US society that takes place in the 2020s because of environmental destruction, wealth inequities, and excessive corporate power. Similarly, Kim Stanley Robinson writes books like *The Ministry for the Future* that imagine how our global society might come to choose different policy solutions to address climate change. These books belong to the genre of speculative fiction, which tells stories that are not based in reality or recorded history but allow us to contemplate alternative futures or directions that our society could take.

Given the vast inequities in our society, speculative fiction that is created by people whose communities have been historically marginalized can help us all to imagine a future that disrupts the inequalities we see in the present day. One example is art and literature from Afro-futurism thought-leaders. Afro-futurism is specifically a branch of literature and other thought that imagines a future where Black people are thriving. It recognizes a traumatic past and present and works to envision a different future. As described by art education professor Dr. Kathy Brown, Afro-futurism is about "forward thinking as well as backward thinking. Having a distressing past, a distressing present, but still looking forward to thriving in the future."[15] This work connects with the Black radical imagination that Robin D. G. Kelley writes about in *Freedom Dreams*.[16] These imagined futures in Afro-futurism and other types of storytelling serve to clarify where the choices of present-day society may lead us and what alternatives may exist.

If we do not use our imagination to envision alternative systems, different laws and norms, and new futures, we can start to think that things are inevitable. It becomes inevitable that some segment of our society will live in poverty and struggle to meet their basic needs. It becomes inevitable that we will pollute the Earth. It becomes inevitable that over a million people need to be imprisoned.

Speculative fiction author Ursula K. Le Guin presciently highlights how our current ways of doing things are not necessarily permanent: "We live in capitalism. Its power seems inescapable. So did the divine right of kings. Any human power can be resisted and changed by human beings."[17]

Sometimes dominant views can cloud our ability to envision alternatives. The "divine right of kings" persisted for so many generations that imagining a time before or after it was difficult. But evolutions and revolutions do occur, and they shift how people think about their behaviors, systems, policies, and institutions.

* * *

Holding an incomplete perspective can cause harm. The very first president of the United States was not killed in a dramatic duel like Alexander Hamilton was. He did not die peacefully in his sleep like Benjamin Franklin, or perish in battle like John Laurens. George Washington was taken out by an incomplete understanding of how the body works. He died from a common illness and a common medical treatment that we now know can be extremely harmful. The story of his death illuminates the harms of decision-making based on a faulty or incomplete perspective.

On a chilly December evening in 1799, George Washington's cold-like symptoms were taking a turn for the worse. George and his wife Martha were hunkered down in their bedroom near a warm fire when he began to have trouble breathing. They called for Dr. James Craik, Washington's friend and physician for over 40 years.

The first tool that Dr. Craik and others caring for the 67-year-old Washington used was bloodletting. Bloodletting is a gruesome procedure where you cut open a vein and let blood flow out of a patient's body. The use of bloodletting has a long history starting with the ancient Egyptians; it was used by the Greeks and Romans as well. Hippocrates, a Greek physician traditionally known as the Father of Medicine, believed that human health was dependent on the four humors: blood, phlegm, black bile, and yellow bile. He argued that illness was caused by an imbalance in these bodily fluids that needed to be corrected. Building on this idea of the four humors, Galen of Pergamum, a prominent second-century Roman physician and philosopher, argued that blood was the most important of the humors, which provided rationale for the practice of removing blood from a patient's body.[18]

Bloodletting could be conducted in various ways, including the use of knives, leeches, or skin scraping. The most common method was to use sharp pointed knives to open up an artery. Physicians sometimes referred to this as "breathing a vein," and it was considered quite simple: removing blood from a patient was supposed to resolve their ailment. For centuries, it was the recommended practice for cancer, cholera, epilepsy, plague, and numerous other health issues. But, as 19th-century science—and 21st-century intuition—would show, bloodletting was not just ineffective at resolving these health issues, it also *harmed* patients.

By the time Washington became the first president of the newly formed United States of America, bloodletting was a common practice for various health issues. So, when he was sick with a throat infection, it was one of the first responses used by Dr. Craik. In fact, bloodletting was so common and widely believed as a cure-all that Washington requested it immediately when he became ill. On that winter evening in December 1799—before the discovery of antibiotics to treat an infection—Washington and his loved ones knew that a throat infection could prove fatal. They feared he would not live to see the dawn of the next century.

In total, Dr. Craik and his team removed blood from Washington four times within the 24 hours before Washington died.[19] It is estimated that the bloodletting removed over half the blood in his body. Several researchers have examined this moment in medical history and determined that the bloodletting was very likely a key cause of his death.

Doctors treated Washington's illness with faulty and harmful solutions—horrifying solutions given what we know now—because of a failure to understand how the human body works. They chose this course of action even though English physician William Harvey, Fellow of the Royal College of Physicians and physician to King James I, conducted research in the 1600s that suggested bloodletting would not work to cure illnesses. And they chose it despite the fact that Charles II, another head of state, died in 1685 after bloodletting. People had been so indoctrinated for centuries about the idea of the "four humors" that even evidence to the contrary did not sway them. It simply *had* to be true that removing blood would heal a patient because it had always been done. Why would people use it if it didn't work?

Thankfully, bloodletting fell out of favor in the late 19th century as the germ theory of disease and improved understanding of the circulatory system took hold. Doctors and the general public began to understand that microscopic germs were the cause of illnesses, not an imbalance in the four humors. People started to shift their idea of how the body worked, paying less attention to an imbalance in bodily fluids and more attention to what germs a patient was exposed to and how. Evidence accumulated and more trusted voices changed their views to fundamentally change how illnesses were treated. Based on new knowledge, doctors and healers began to think about how to *prevent* people from being exposed to germs in the first place.

Reforming or making small modifications to bloodletting practices would have been futile in improving patient outcomes because they were based on faulty beliefs about how the human body worked. Maybe Washington would not have died if they took two liters of blood instead of four, but no matter what tweaks to the approach were made, it would still harm patients in some way. Instead, medical and public health professionals responsible for keeping people healthy had to completely transform how they thought about treatments. With a better understanding of how the body worked, they could better make decisions about how to treat the patient.

Fast-forward to 2019, when I had a persistent sore throat and visited my doctor. She swabbed my throat, did a culture, and determined that I had a throat infection caused by group *A Streptococcus*. It could be treated with a medicine, antibiotics, that had been discovered in the 20th century because of our new understanding of germs. Gratefully, I kept all the blood in my body and my condition improved quickly. This new and improved understanding of how disease and the human body worked—the germ theory of disease—made it all possible.

* * *

If we turn our attention away from individual patients who are suffering and think about our society, we need a new theory of how to stop suffering and allow all people in our society to thrive. We are stuck in old ways of thinking that are not up to date with the latest evidence on what allows people to thrive. Responding to harmful ailments of the human body is analogous to responding to harmful ailments of the body politic. Our public policies and budget allocations are the "treatments" or responses that we give to the body politic when it is suffering from ailments such as violence, homelessness, illness, climate change, poverty, and economic depression.

But are the policies that we currently use based on a faulty understanding of how our society works? Are we failing to see the water simply because we have never let ourselves imagine dry land? Are we clinging to systems and policies that were developed before we had more sophisticated knowledge of how human societies can thrive? To what extent are our outdated ideas and policy treatments actually *causing harm*? And can we *prevent* these bad things from happening in the first place?

When we take a closer look at our current policies and systems, using a critical eye and our imagination, we open up new possibilities to transform our society at the roots.

CHAPTER 2

Roots

In the course of history, there comes a time when humanity is called to shift to a new level of consciousness, to reach a higher moral ground. A time when we have to shed our fear and give hope to each other. That time is now.
—Kenyan activist and Nobel Peace Prize winner Wangarī Maathai

Mari Copeny is a child of the 21st century, and her life has been shaped by the public policy decisions by the "grown-ups" in the room. She was born in 2007, and her life would likely have been very different had she not been born in Flint, Michigan. A few months before her seventh birthday, a man appointed by the governor of Michigan decided to change Flint's water supply from the vast freshwater Lake Huron to the polluted Flint River.

This type of decision on municipal water supply would ordinarily be a public policy decision by the democratically elected Flint city council. Instead, that decision was made by a state-appointed "emergency manager" because of 2012 legislation in Michigan targeting Michigan municipalities that were struggling financially. The emergency manager had no accountability to the residents of Flint, only to Michigan's governor. In the haste to save money, the emergency manager and officials failed to apply corrosion inhibitors to the polluted water supply, which resulted in lead being released from aging pipes within Flint. This was the most immediate policy decision that led to Mari and other Flint children experiencing harmful lead exposure.[20] Exposure like this at such a young age can cause slowed growth and development, learning and behavior problems, and hearing and speech problems.

The decision by the emergency manager to change the water source stemmed from policy decisions made decades earlier.[20] In the 20th century, public policies at various levels shaped Flint into what it is today and created the conditions for the present-day disaster. Economic policies prioritized corporate profit, which facilitated the closure of the General Motors car factory and ultimately led to widespread unemployment or underemployment. This caused a drop in municipal income taxes, which was accompanied by a decrease in property taxes and state-level policies that reduced revenue-sharing from the state government. In a parallel development, incarceration policies in Michigan locked up an increasing number of residents—disproportionately Black—which severely limited their ability to contribute to their community or the tax base.[21] A combination of transportation, housing, education, and economic policies created sprawl and increased racial segregation, ultimately leading to Flint being a majority Black city. Majority Black cities struggle to attract investment and growth because of the racism baked into our financial institutions and discrimination by white people who avoid living, visiting, or working in such settings. The economic distress on Flint's budget, caused by all these policies, led directly to the imposition of an emergency manager and ultimately the Flint water crisis.

Flint's emergency manager expected to save $5 million by switching the city's water source. What actually followed was an infamous water crisis that caused thousands of children like Mari to experience lead poisoning. Compounding this tragedy,

12 people died from Legionnaire's disease. The health damages from the Flint water crisis have already cost taxpayers more than $600 million and is likely to cost much more in the future.[22]

This is the context and backdrop of Mari's youth: a legacy of failed public policies that have prioritized corporate profit and the comfort of white residents over policies that would help the entire community thrive. You can contrast that with the context of my own youth. I grew up as a resident of a predominantly white suburb of Chicago with well-funded public schools, safe water, and a robust tax base of middle-class and upper-class professionals. As a youth, I focused my attention on winning soccer games, hanging out with friends, and getting into college. Residents from my town were the beneficiaries of corporate profits and were not the targets of incarceration policies. Even if my town had been struggling financially, I doubt the governor would have felt it was prudent to usurp power from our democratically elected decision-makers and appoint an emergency manager. People like me derived advantages from the same policies that caused harm in Mari's community.

My community and Mari's community are unequal. There are differences between them. One had more abundant resources and the other had fewer. But they are not just unequal—they are *inequitable*. An inequity means the inequality is the result of an injustice. The inequality between our two communities is not just due to chance or an accident. An inequity is an inequality that is both unfair *and avoidable*. In other words, it does not have to be this way. But our decisions as a society have made it this way.

For many people, public policies are largely invisible. In day-to-day life, we often forget that the roads in our neighborhood and the types of houses or stores available are the results of policy choices. Zoning policies determine what types of houses can be built (apartments versus duplexes versus single-family homes) or what types of businesses can be established. Transportation policies determine where roads will go, how many lanes they will have, what the speed limit is, whether the roads have bike lanes, and what type of vehicles are allowed to use them. It can be the difference between a neighborhood divided by a major highway or a pedestrian-friendly small street. These examples are largely determined at the local level; federal and state policies can have an even bigger impact.

State-level policy decisions determine that schools must be funded at the local level based on a local tax base. That guaranteed that the public schools I went to as a child were well-resourced, and it guaranteed that the public schools in Flint were underfunded. As a kid, I was aware that schools could be unequal, but I did not fully comprehend the *inequities* or how those inequities could be caused by public policies. I was able to drift through my childhood without giving much attention to the public policies shaping my life chances.

Mari did not have the same privilege to ignore policies. Those policies upended her life at an early age. But she did not just stand idly by and watch them harm her community. She has taken action to push policymakers to reenvision different public policies. Mari says, "My generation will fix this mess. Watch us."[23]

Mari is now a leading national activist fighting against public policies that neglect the needs of communities like Flint. In 2016, she wrote a letter to President Barack Obama explaining the urgent situation in Flint and imploring him to visit.[24] This helped lead to President Obama traveling to Flint and ultimately pledging a $80 million aid package to help address the crisis.[25] While this budget allocation and subsequent funding may help to mitigate to harms that have already occurred, Mari is working in other cities across the country to advocate for public policies that can prevent such harms *before they happen.*

Mari understands that our decisions as a society affect who lives, who dies, and who thrives. Policies at the federal, state, and local level are attempting to address societal ills and build a functioning society. The policy to change the water source was trying to solve the municipal budget crisis. Because of ignorance and negligence, it had severe negative consequences beyond its intended purpose. It was not trying to address the root cause of the municipal budget crisis; it was merely responding to one of its symptoms.

Making the wrong policy choice can have a far-reaching and permanent impact on the lives of not just one individual but potentially thousands or millions of people. For the Flint water crisis, the root of the problem stemmed from the history that preceded it. The roots were the policies that enabled racial discrimination and privileged profits over the needs of human residents.

* * *

Policymakers too often make decisions that put us in what I call the public policy paradox.[26] We saw it in Flint, and we will see other examples of it throughout this book. The paradox is that our governments spend a lot of money—or deprive communities of money—which ultimately causes harm in some way. Then, that same government funds the services needed to clean up the mess. We see examples in so many different areas. We spend a lot of money on things that research shows harms communities in the name of safety (e.g., prisons). We allow other harms in the name of profit (e.g., pollution) and deprive communities of resources in the name of cost-savings (e.g., clean water, school funding).

Then, we have entire government agencies with dedicated funding aimed at improving health, improving educational outcomes, and addressing poverty. The US Department of Health and Human Services had a fiscal year 2024 budget of $144 billion in discretionary spending (and $1.7 trillion in mandatory spending on things like Medicare and Medicaid) to address issues related to health and poverty that were in part caused by the policy failures of our criminal legal system, educational system, and environmental protection policies.[27] This is our paradox. We spend vast amounts of money on public policies that we know cause problems while simultaneously funding agencies to fix those problems.

These policy decisions have a huge impact on our health and well-being. This has been well documented in rigorous research and in the excellent book *The Political Determinants of Health* by Daniel Dawes.[28] Simply put, our policy choices are life or death.

We should not ignore the fact that policies that have contributed to harm are not merely accidents. In many cases, powerful people have lobbied for policies that would harm others in order to secure their own wealth and safety.[29]

With all of these policy choices, we are doing the equivalent of bloodletting our society. We are choosing treatments for our body politic that have been shown to be harmful overall and particularly harmful for people of color and other marginalized groups. The conventional wisdom is that we have access to the best health care in the world, that our education policies create a meritocracy, that our environmental policies will promote economic prosperity, and that our criminal legal system makes us all safer. But this conventional wisdom is not supported by the scientific evidence, just like bloodletting was not supported by scientific evidence. And, crucially, it is not supported by the personal experience of people living in poor and disadvantaged communities.

We need to imagine doing better. Our policy choices are in some cases extremely costly and ineffective—and sometimes extremely harmful—at creating a society where everyone has the opportunity to thrive. Our policy choices are often leading to the very problems we theoretically want to prevent. Doing better will require creating a future where our public policies address the root causes of societal problems.

* * *

Irving Zola was a medical sociologist and activist who helped to found the field of disability studies. His work turned the lens away from individuals and focused on how the broader environment and policy landscape shaped people's ability to thrive. He is credited with a famous parable—frequently used in the field of public health—about the importance of identifying solutions that get at the root of a problem. While it has many iterations, Zola said:

> There I am standing by the shore of a swiftly flowing river, and I hear the cry of a drowning man. So I jump into the river, put my arms around him, pull him to shore, and apply artificial respiration. Just when he begins to breathe, there is another cry for help. So I jump into the river, reach him, pull him to shore, apply artificial respiration, and then just as he begins to breathe, another cry for help. So back in the river again, reaching, pulling, applying, breathing, and then another yell. Again and again, without end, goes the sequence. You know, I am so busy jumping in, pulling them to shore, applying artificial respiration, that I have no time to see who the hell is upstream pushing them all in.

In some versions, people are falling in the river upstream because of a crumbling bridge or a lack of signage about a dangerous river. Another version implies that a corporation is making money off people jumping in the river. In all of these cases, the point is that we need to seek out the *root cause* of the problem. We can and do spend a tremendous amount of energy responding to a problem, but we will be much more efficient if we tackle the root cause.

This parable prompts us to think about where we are dedicating our energy and resources. For example, an examination of our current health care system would show that we spend vast amount of resources rescuing drowning people from the river and not enough addressing upstream causes to see what could prevent them from drowning in the first place.

I teach my public health students to ask questions to help them dig deeper and identify the root cause of an issue. Using the parable described as an example, digging deeper goes a little something like this:

Q: *Why are there people drowning in the river?*
A: They are in this part of the river that is very fast flowing.

Q: *Why are they in that dangerous part of the river?*
A: The current took them from further upstream.

Q: *Why did they go in the water further upstream?*
A: Someone pushed them in.

Q: *Why did that person push them in?*
A: They just stole their wallet and didn't want to get caught.

Q: *Why did they steal their wallet?*
A: They don't have any money for their rent payment and were worried their family would get evicted.

Q: *Why don't they have any money?*
A: They work a full-time minimum wage job, but that still doesn't cover basic needs.

Q: *Why doesn't minimum wage cover basic human needs?*
A: Special interest groups have prevented politicians from raising minimum wages, and we have an inadequate social safety net to supplement that minimum wage.

We could keep digging deeper and uncover issues like unregulated capitalism, voter suppression tactics, neoliberalism, and campaign finance laws. If you don't ask enough questions, you do not get to the root causes of an issue.

If a community wanted to address the river drowning issue in this town, there are any number of policy solutions they could take. If they just asked the initial question, they might decide that the solution is to staff lifeguards at the river bank. They might also build a rope for people to grab onto as they floated by, or they could implement widespread swimming lessons. Perhaps the community is wise enough to move beyond the first question and ask a few follow-ups. They might look further upstream and identify that person who is pushing people in is the problem. They might try to tackle that problem with a police presence or by creating harsh punishments. But if we just keep digging deeper, we would realize that our community has created conditions that are encouraging people to steal and push people into the river. Obviously, pushing people into the river is a huge societal problem. But if we can view it not as a moral shortcoming of one individual but instead a deficiency of our whole society that creates conditions that motivate people to behave this way, then we come to very different conclusions about how to address the problem. We need to dig deep enough to see the roots to really identify the structures and policies that are in place that create conditions for harm.

In the field of public health, we focus on creating programs or policies that will *prevent* bad outcomes and hopefully promote good outcomes, and we describe three types of prevention: primary, secondary, and tertiary. Primary prevention is when you are able to stop the health issue from occurring in the first place. Basically, the person never is in the river in the first place. Secondary prevention usually refers to screening for a health issue so that you catch it at the earliest possible time and can effectively treat or mitigate its harms. Maybe you have a crew set up before the river's rapids get strong to stop people in the river from continuing to real dangerous territory. You can think about screenings for cancer or household lead exposure, commonly used in an attempt to catch the issue before it gets worse. Finally, tertiary prevention mostly refers to slowing disease progression with treatment. The river might have a rope where people in the river can hang on and either save themselves or delay their drowning. Tertiary prevention often refers to solutions that make a health issue less bad, like taking pain relievers for a migraine or chemotherapy after being diagnosed with cancer.

Thinking about the three types of prevention, which one would you allocate the most resources toward? If you agree with the World Health Organization and other prominent health institutions, you would want to focus your energies and resources on primary prevention: trying to stop the health issue before it ever started. But the reality is that our governmental health resources in the United States are overwhelmingly spent on tertiary prevention and somewhat on secondary prevention. We focus our health resources mostly on treating people who are already sick.

If we broaden our lens a bit to think about these types of prevention outside the context of health, where are most of our policies aimed? When our government spends money on people without housing, do we try and prevent them from being homeless in the first place, or do we try and give them resources to cope with being homeless? How about poverty? Do we try to prevent corporations from paying poverty wages, or do we just provide a few small resources to the people who experience poverty wages? What about violence? Do we focus more resources on trying to prevent the violence from ever happening or on trying to stop it after it has already happened? Think about food insecurity. Do we try to ensure that everyone can afford and access enough food, or do we give financial aid to people who are experiencing food insecurity so that it doesn't get worse? As a society, we tend to wait for the bad things to happen, and then we throw some resources at it to try and make it a little less bad. But ultimately, the violence and food insecurity and poverty occurred. If we are serious about addressing these harms, we would spend money to prevent them from happening in the first place.

A key part of preventing things before they happen is asking the people directly affected about what they need. A common phrase within marginalized communities advocating for the resources they deserve is "nothing about us without us." This means that decisions about what type of primary prevention we should adopt should be made with the impacted communities at the center of the decision-making. Somebody who is food insecure can tell you that their minimum wage job simply does not cover the grocery bill or their Social Security check does not cover the bills. Because they are living it, they can point out the root cause of the issue. Government policymaking is less effective and less preventative when impacted communities are not engaged and empowered to identify solutions.

In 2022, the *New York Times* published an article about the state of type 2 diabetes prevention and treatment with an accompanying tweet that said: "Researchers who study Type 2 diabetes have reached a stark conclusion: There is no device or drug powerful enough to counter the effects of poverty, pollution, stress, a broken food system, cities that aren't walkable, and inequitable access to healthcare."[30] The tweet made it seem as if this was a new discovery. But, people who have considered the river parable and dug deep to examine root causes have long known that a medical device or a drug is just like the person trying to go in and save the drowning person. Ultimately, the drug might save the person, but don't we want them to avoid drowning or getting diabetes in the first place? Upstream factors—or the "poverty, pollution, stress, a broken food system, cities that aren't walkable, and inequitable access to healthcare," as the *New York Times* describes them—are so much more crucial to diabetes outcomes. And this isn't true of just diabetes. It is true of all health issues. Simply put, study after study shows that the way we have built our society is bad for our collective health and ability to thrive.[31-33]

* * *

Our culture puts a lot of emphasis on the quick fix or a pill that can solve our problems. But those who study many of these issues have thoroughly critiqued that idea. Bruce Link and Jo Phelan are two health researchers who observed that a lot of research was focused on an extremely narrow aspect of the "cause" of a problem. In their field, research was directed toward "risk factors" for a specific disease. Diabetes researchers were looking at risk factors like diet and exercise; HIV researchers were looking at risk factors like condom use and the number of sexual partners. But Link and Phelan recognized that much of this work was merely focused on that *swiftly flowing river* and not on the person pushing people in the river.[34]

The research looked at the immediate cause, rather than the conditions that caused it. When researchers were looking at diabetes deaths, they were mostly zeroing in on an individual's behaviors and not the condition that our society created to either promote or create barriers to healthy behaviors. Diet and exercise are not solely about individual choices without consideration of the broader environment. A person's food and exercise choices are shaped by whether they live and work in an environment that promotes physical activity, whether they have access to healthy foods, and whether their other basic needs are met so that they can spend energy on exercise and a healthy diet. A person earning minimum wage while living in an unsafe neighborhood where no grocery stores exist will have vastly different opportunities for good diet and exercise routines than a salaried person living in a well-resourced suburb near a fully stocked grocery store. Individual choices certainly play a role, but the conditions that shape these choices are a crucial component.

The Fundamental Cause Theory developed by Link and Phelan points to the structures and policies that create conditions for thriving or creates conditions for harm. The theory draws the attention away from an individual's choices and behaviors and instead turns the lens on the systems, policies, and norms that give people access to resources like power, money, prestige, and knowledge. When we talk about getting at the root cause of an issue, it is these *fundamental causes* that we need to tackle and transform.

So, what does this all mean for how we start transforming at the root to address problems in our society and shift public policies in our country? It means that we need a *prevention mindset* to help us stop problems before they start rather than seeking the quick-fix pill that will solve it after the fact. A prevention mindset means we need to:

1. Identify the root causes of a problem (e.g., keep digging deeper).
2. Prioritize primary prevention (e.g., stop bad things from happening in the first place).
3. Focus prevention on what the impacted group wants and needs (e.g., nothing about us without us).

This prevention mindset—a term that I will return to throughout the book—can help us get at the root of problems. It will also prompt many hard questions for our society. Once we start looking into root causes of many issues, we are likely to identify the economic system or political system or criminal legal system in the United States as a key contributing factor. We often hear big, transformative policy proposals shouted down as radical. But, as Angela Davis reminds us, "Radical simply means 'grasping things at the root.'"[35] The word *radical* comes from the Latin words "radic" or "radicalis," which simply means "roots." Being radical may be exactly what we need to put this prevention mindset into practice.

What gets labeled as radical policies may not actually be that radical. After all, think about the river parable. Which sounds more radical: spending billions of dollars on life preservers to help drowning people or spending billions to ensure no one gets pushed in the river in the first place? Which is more radical: prioritizing the ideas of the CEO of the life preserver company or listening to the people who are most likely to be pushed in the river? Using a prevention mindset will help us get at the roots and more efficiently and effectively create public policy solutions.

Part II of this book will invite us to reflect on our public policy choices in different areas—health care, public safety, criminal legal system, environment, and education—in order to apply a prevention mindset and imagine what doing better could look like.

PART II

Reflection

CHAPTER 3

Better Health Care

Is Health Care Like Kindergarten or Like Soybeans?

Xiomara, a Nicaraguan woman in her mid-50s, was a true revolutionary, someone who was part of her country's revolution to overthrow a dictator and establish a society founded on principles of fairness and equity. I met and befriended Xiomara when I was a Peace Corps volunteer and worked at a government-operated local health center that provided primary care and prevention services for a town of about 20,000. I was assigned to work alongside Xiomara, who was in charge of community outreach for the health center.

Xiomara and I were working and living in one of the hottest parts of the country, so our most important workplace accessory was a sweat rag to wipe our brows. Together, we went into schools, led youth groups, weighed babies, and participated in door-to-door vaccination campaigns (among other health promotion activities). During the hottest part of the day, we'd take a break, sometimes buying a glass-bottle Coca-Cola or homemade fresh fruit juice cleverly served in a small, clear plastic bag tied around a straw. She would regale me with stories of the revolution and lovingly refer to me as a *yanqui imperialista*.

Xiomara was employed by the government, as were all of our colleagues at the health center. The health center was part of the government's guarantee of health for its residents. The government and residents viewed health as a fundamental human right. Politics and policies in Nicaragua have changed quite a bit over the past decade, but when I was there, the government-run clinic provided free universal health care coverage for all residents. Residents could walk into any clinic and be seen by a medical professional. No insurance cards. No billing department. Every town had at least one health center that provided both basic medical care and community outreach for programs like vaccines and health education.

Nicaragua was, and still is, a relatively poor country without many resources. There were limitations on the services that they could provide freely to all residents. But health was viewed as a fundamental human right, similar to how we view a right to K-12 education in the United States. The government and residents believed it would be too cruel, and a violation of a human right, to deny someone health care simply because they did not have enough money. In the United States, most people would agree that it would be cruel and a violation of a human right to deny a child the ability to enroll in kindergarten simply because their family did not have enough money.

Xiomara and my other Nicaraguan friends and colleagues would talk about differences in how we view health in the United States compared to Nicaragua. At the time, I knew the US health care system was not perfect, but before living in Nicaragua, I had not yet fully understood the distinction between health as a human right and health as a commodity. But Xiomara and the Nicaraguans I worked with saw this clearly. They would ask me: "How can you trust a doctor who could make more money depending on what they recommend to you?" I had never thought of it that way, but they made an interesting point. Especially in a private practice or other settings, doctors could make more money if they recommended a certain procedure or medication (even aside from the possible kickbacks for prescribing certain medications).[36]

They were also very curious about hypothetical situations in the United States. For instance, "What would someone do if they needed medication urgently but couldn't afford it?" or "What happens if someone gets in an accident but doesn't have insurance or money?" Because I had always had health coverage through my parents' insurance plan or the Peace Corps, I had never fully wrestled with or experienced these hypotheticals. Now that I work in public health with many poor and marginalized communities, I hear about these real-life stories frequently. I now know that they are not just hypotheticals. Medical expenses cause more than half of all bankruptcies in this country.[37]

* * *

In the United States, there is no guarantee you can receive health services. While we do have subsidies or programs for some people who are struggling financially, not everyone gets this support. Emergency rooms are not allowed to turn away people for lack of payment, but emergency rooms are mostly oriented toward stopping an emergency rather than helping you become healthy. If you are poor or lower-middle class, you simply might not be able to afford primary health care in the United States. In contrast, the perspective that health is a human right holds that anyone should be able to have their health needs addressed, regardless of how much money they have (or any other factors). Many countries across the world consider health to be a fundamental human right. But it is not our approach in US policy.

According to the World Health Organization, health is "a state of complete physical, mental and social well-being and not merely the absence of disease or infirmity." Health as a human right does not mean that everyone in a society is guaranteed to be healthy, only that everyone has the opportunity to be healthy.[38] If you craft public policies with the idea that health is a human right, you guarantee medical care for everyone and take care of physical, mental, and social well-being.

In the United States, we have taken a different path. Our public policies largely view health and health care as commodities.[39,40] Medical appointments, exams, medications, healthy foods, opportunities for exercise, and mental health and other services are not guaranteed or provided by the government; rather, individuals largely have to purchase such services with their own money (or pay an insurance company to pay for it). A commodity is a resource that can be exchanged for a resource that has a similar value. In the United States, we typically exchange health care that we receive for money. Other examples of commodities are soybeans, clothing, or gas. Sacks of soybeans are like medical services in the United States—they have a cost, and someone must be able to pay that cost in order to have that service (or those soybeans). Many people have some form of health insurance that pays for their health services. Some employers compensate employees with health insurance instead of paying them a higher salary. There is some public funding and subsidies for health care (e.g., Medicaid, Medicare, health insurance exchanges), but those resources are not available to everyone.

* * *

The idea of health as a human right was established in the tumult of the years at the end of World War II. Many countries were reeling and in shock by the atrocities committed against humans. In this aftermath, countries came together to form the United Nations (UN) and began working on developing norms, policies, and institutions that could prevent future harms. They were thinking with a prevention mindset: How do we create a world where this can never happen again?

In April 1945, thousands of delegates from 50 nations descended on San Francisco for the UN Conference on International Organization. This meeting would ultimately establish the first UN Charter and set many other initiatives in motion. Imagine the scene: people from all over the world, speaking different languages, trying to figure out what the new global order would look like. What institutions would they need? What values would they enshrine in policy? How would they make decisions? So much of what followed in 20th-century world governance was debated at that conference.

At this conference, three delegates who were doctors—Szeming Sze (China), Paula Souza (Brazil), and Karl Evang (Norway)—were trying to ensure that nations came together to establish an international health organization. They first tried to submit an amendment to the new UN charter, but it was too late. Then they tried to get one of the formal committees to take it up, but it got stuck there. Finally, during a chance dinner meeting with the secretary general of the conference, Dr. Sze received critical advice: the best way of getting the health organization established was through a declaration. The declaration was passed with overwhelming support and led to the establishment of the World Health Organization (WHO) the following year as an offshoot of the UN.[41] In 1946, the WHO drafted its first constitution, which established "the highest attainable standard of health as a fundamental right of every human being without distinction of race, religion, political belief, economic or social condition."[42]

At the same time that the WHO was writing health as a human right into its constitution, another part of the emerging UN was trying to gain international agreement on fundamental human rights. In 1946, former US first lady Eleanor Roosevelt became chair of the commission that was tasked by the UN General Assembly with writing a declaration on human rights that all member nations could agree to. Eleanor Roosevelt took this charge extremely seriously, hoping that crafting a unanimous declaration would help prevent future wars or atrocities like the Holocaust. And this was all taking place during the start of the Cold War with Soviet–US tensions running high.[43]

Roosevelt chaired over 3,000 hours of deliberations where delegates from around the world ultimately agreed on 30 articles to the UN Declaration on Human Rights. All 192 member states of the UN have signed onto the document; with over 500 translations, it has set the Guinness World Record for most translated document.[44]

Importantly, the declaration helped to further establish the idea of health as a human right as the global standard. Article 25 states: *"Everyone has the right to a standard of living adequate for the health and well-being of himself and of his family, including food, clothing, housing and medical care and necessary social services, and the right to security in the event of unemployment, sickness, disability, widowhood, old age or other lack of livelihood in circumstances beyond his control."*[45]

* * *

At this point, all 192 member nations of the UN, including the United States, have signed onto this declaration. But health as a human right has been translated into policy in many different ways across the globe. A literal reading of this human right would indicate that a nation-state needs to guarantee food, clothing, housing, medical care, and other necessary social services to its residents. Some countries have taken this seriously by providing universal health care *and* expansive social services. For example, Scandinavian countries have universal health care coverage accompanied by a robust social safety net that provides food, shelter, and other needed goods for people who cannot pay for it themselves.

All the wealthy industrialized nations except for the United States provide universal health care for everyone in their society.[46] Countries with fewer resources are a mixed bag. Some (like Nicaragua) have still adopted a universal coverage ethos even if limited funding means that the execution of this ethos leaves gaps in services. Low-resource countries often struggle to provide comprehensive care and may have strict limitations on what type of care is included.

In the United States, we have fallen quite short of this human rights declaration.[47] US public policy has made access to health care a commodity. It is a privilege and not a right. While you can pay out of pocket for health care in the United States, most people pay a health insurance company (either directly or their employer pays); the insurer then pays health care costs. Well, sort of. Health insurance companies pay costs after you have already paid some costs (a deductible), and they put maximum limits on how much they will cover (a cap). A minority of Americans get their health insurance through government programs such as Medicaid or Medicare, or they receive health care at no cost through government-funded health care facilities like the Veterans Administration or federally qualified health centers. But this patchwork leaves many behind and creates some serious bureaucratic nightmares.

In 2023, about 9% of Americans ages 0–64 did not have health insurance.[48] Medicaid provides health care coverage for low-income Americans, but state policies can place severe eligibility restrictions. In some states, adults without children or without disabilities are not eligible at all, regardless of their income level. The Affordable Care Act tried to expand eligibility for Medicaid across the country, but—as of 2024—10 states have made the decision to opt out, despite federal funding to support the expansion (several states made the decision to opt in years after initially opting out).[49]

In states that did not expand Medicaid eligibility, low-income adults without dependent children are simply not eligible for this government-funded health insurance, and that has life-and-death consequences. Texas was one of the states that made a choice to not expand Medicaid coverage. In the initial years since opting out, researchers estimate that about 2,900 Texans ages 55–64 died due to that policy choice. They would have still been alive if Texas had opted in.[50] Thousands of families lost a loved one, workplaces lost a colleague, and communities lost a neighbor all because Texan policymakers chose to make health care a commodity that some people could not access. Those 2,900 deaths are roughly the same number of people who died on September 11, 2001.

In contrast, there are an estimated 19,000 people across the United States who were alive in 2022 only because they were lucky enough to live in one of the 33 states that expanded Medicaid coverage.[50] If you live in one of the Medicaid expansion states, it is very possible that one of your family members, neighbors, kid's teachers, colleagues, or friends is alive today because they were able to access health services through the Medicaid expansion.

*   *   *

Even for those of us lucky enough to have health insurance, our system is set up to discourage us from receiving needed health care. In 2022, my doctor advised me to get a colonoscopy because of my persistent gastrointestinal issues. Aside from the challenges of taking a day off from work and finding transportation, this procedure—not elective, it was recommended by my primary care physician—was quite costly. The hospital charged me $6,732, and my excellent employer-paid insurance covered $5,844, leaving me with an out-of-pocket bill of $889. Frankly, if I had realized how much I would have to pay out of pocket, I might have opted not to do it, even though I can technically afford that amount. Think of all the fun things I could have done with $889 instead of getting a colonoscopy. If that choice would have been presented to me, I probably would have chosen to avoid it or delay it.

Now, compare those costs to the expense of a colonoscopy if I lived just 45 miles away from my home in Michigan and across the border into Canada. Under the health care policies of Canada, the *total* cost of the procedure would have been less than $500.[51] That is less than 10% of the $6,732 that my hospital in Michigan charged me. And how much would I have had to pay out of pocket? Zero dollars. The entire cost of the procedure (less than $500!) would have been fully covered by Canadian taxpayers through their government-funded health care system.

My $889 out-of-pocket expense needs to be considered next to the statistic that 40% of Americans say they would struggle to pay for an unexpected $400 expense.[52] Do you think they would have gotten the colonoscopy if they were in my situation? Thankfully, my procedure found nothing serious, but it easily could have provided an early diagnosis of colon cancer or prevented another serious illness. Unfortunately, our health care system—built on a foundation of public policies—has incentivized people to *avoid* health care services until it is too late.

Let us return to the fact that medical expenses account for more than half of all bankruptcies.[37] Think about what that means. If you have the misfortune to be in an accident or diagnosed with a severe issue, it is going to be very expensive. This is usually true even for people with "good" health insurance. Some folks can weather this expense because they have savings, wealthy family members, or good-paying jobs. But most people have limited resources to cope with these costs.

How many times has a GoFundMe page related to medical expenses come across your social media accounts or email? I would bet that most readers have even donated to a friend or family member who was collecting money to help pay their medical expenses. Medical expenses contribute to more than 500,000 bankruptcies in the United States *per year*. Fundraisers for medical expenses is an entire category on GoFundMe, and there are even resources to show people how to create these campaigns. According to GoFundMe, it hosts more than 250,000 fundraisers for personal medical expenses a year and raises $650 million annually. But a recent study showed that most of them failed to collect the needed expenses.[53] So, while GoFundMe and other crowdsourcing tactics can help people pay for medical expenses, most people are unable to solve their issue this way.

* * *

Our current commodity-based health care system is a root cause of the deaths and financial ruin of some people. But it is important to note that these harms are not distributed equally across society. As you can imagine, they disproportionately affect poor Americans. About 80% of people who are uninsured have an income that puts them below 400% of the poverty line.[54] In 2021, for an individual, below 400% of the poverty line would mean earning less than $51,520 annually.

Because the United States is a deeply racialized society, these harms are also patterned by race. People from racially marginalized groups are more likely to be uninsured: 21% of American Indians/Alaska Natives, 21% of Native Hawaiians/Pacific Islanders, 19% of Latinos, and 11% of Black Americans are uninsured compared to only 7% of whites.[54] About 28% of Black households and 22% of Hispanic households had medical debt that they could not pay, compared to about 17% for white households.[55]

So how does this deeply unequal commodity-based system stack up in terms of overall spending and health outcomes compared to other wealthy countries that take a "health as human right" approach?[56] Well, the percentage that the United States spends on health care as a share of its economy is more than twice the average of other nations in the Organization for Economic Cooperation and Development (OECD). Compared with 10 other high-income countries that all have government-sponsored universal health care, the United States had the lowest life expectancy, highest suicide rates, highest chronic disease burden, highest number of hospitalizations from preventable causes, and highest rate of avoidable deaths.[56] It is hardly a ringing endorsement for a commodity-based system for health care.

Imagining a Better World: Policies Based on a Prevention Mindset

How can we take a prevention mindset to this issue? If we look at the root causes of poor health outcomes, we do not even have to dig that deep in this instance. Simply, our health care system is preventing people from receiving care. We could dig deeper to find out why people are needing health care services in the first place (something later chapters will cover), but the most immediate cause of the deaths and medical bankruptcies are not providing universal health care coverage for all residents in the United States. It is as if there is someone handing out life preservers to drowning people downstream, except that these life preservers cost $3,000 and most people need a GoFundMe account to afford them.

We think of health care as something to buy and sell, like a sack of soybeans, rather than something everyone has a right to, like children's education. With health care, we thankfully have many other models we can look to across the world since we are the only wealthy nation that has chosen to treat our health care system like soybeans rather than like kindergarten. There are several variations to provide universal health care coverage that are important to note, including a single-payer system and a government-sponsored health system.

The current system in the United States is a multi-payer system where there are various insurance companies, government entities, and individuals who are paying for medical services. In contrast, a single-payer system would shift the equation so that all essential health services were paid for by a single entity, typically government-sponsored insurance. For example, all Canadians have "Medicare," which is paid for by the Canadian government and fully covers needed health expenses. This system is more advantageous than multi-payer because a single entity can more effectively negotiate prices with providers or pharmaceutical companies than a patchwork of smaller companies or entities. That brings overall health care costs down from the stratosphere and is ultimately why services like a colonoscopy in Canada costs less than 10% of what the same procedure costs in the United States.

If you are over age 65 or otherwise qualify for Medicare in the United States, you are covered by a version of the single-payer model. All medical services for that age group are essentially paid for by the same entity: the US government. That is why the leading push for a single-payer system in the United States is called "Medicare for All." The proposal would expand Medicare eligibility to include all US residents. That means that people would no longer receive health insurance paid for by employers or paid through the Affordable Care Act marketplace—they would simply be covered by Medicare automatically. This would dramatically cut health care costs, eliminate most medical bankruptcies, and cut down on inequities related to who can access health care in this country.

There is another iteration of the single-payer health system where the government is not only the payer but also runs the hospitals and clinics as well. An example is the United Kingdom's National Health Service. There, health care providers and all other clinic or hospital staff are government employees. There are some wonderful synergies here since there is no need to negotiate prices or have teams of employees doing this work. All the resources can go into providing patient care.

As a useful analogy, the UK National Health Service is a lot like the public school system in United States, where the government both funds schools and is in charge of staffing and operating them. Teachers are government employees, and schools are typically owned by the government. In contrast, a single-payer system would be like the government paying private school tuition for all children in the country. In this scenario, the government would be the "single payer," but the education would be provided by a nongovernment entity like a private school. While there may be some advantages to such a system, it would likely cost more and be harder to maintain standards of education. The National Health Service has certain efficiencies because it both pays for and provides services. In addition, it is less dependent on private entities to provide adequate care. It gives the government, and ultimately the citizens who fund and vote on the government, greater control over where services are provided and the standards of care.

Much negativity is attached to any discussion of universal health care or a single-payer system in the United States. Many people think it is too radical. Critics say it would result in longer wait times or poorer quality care, but those ideas have been debunked by looking at places where these models have been implemented.[57] It is true that in countries with universal health care, service is rarely delivered perfectly, and some citizens in those countries still have complaints. When comparing those imperfect systems to our own imperfect system, however, those that provide universal coverage spend less money and get better outcomes across the population.

If you study the history of health care in the United States, the reason we do not have single-payer or universal health care has little to do with diminished quality of care. Rather, it has to do with the profits that doctors and insurance companies are able to make. The American Medical Association has fiercely opposed a single-payer system over the past decades—despite the benefits to their patients—largely because it could lower profits earned by doctors.[58]

*   *   *

Universal health care coverage is essential for reducing the worst outcomes of death, illness, medical bankruptcy, and inequities. But it is only a portion of the equation. Health care usually treats health issues after they occur, but a prevention mindset would aim to *prevent* them before they happen. We can look to Costa Rica as an example of a country that has effectively incorporated a prevention mindset into its health care system. In 2019, life expectancy in Costa Rica was 80 years compared to 79 years in the United States, despite Costa Rica only spending $922 per person per year on health care compared to US spending of $10,921 per person per year.[59] What's their secret?

In 2021, noted doctor and health care expert Atul Gawande went searching for an answer to that exact question. In a *New Yorker* article from that year, he concluded:

> The country has made public health—measures to improve the health of the population as a whole—central to the delivery of medical care. Even in countries with robust universal health care, public health is usually an add-on; the vast majority of spending goes to treat the ailments of individuals. In Costa Rica, though, public health has been a priority for decades.[60]

In other words, medical care is only part of the equation for good health. Access to preventative measures that are well integrated into the health care system are essential for promoting good health and longevity.

What does this mean, practically speaking? It means that the health care system should not only focus on patient health but also on the health of the entire surrounding community. A clinic or hospital would not wait for patients to call them to set up a flu shot; instead, they would be visiting their patients' homes, local employers, or otherwise making it easy for their community to prevent disease through flu shots. The current US health care system is not set up for that because the financial incentive is not there. It is set up for patients to come to medical providers and define what their medical needs are, rather than for doctors and clinics to try to prevent those issues before they happen.

In Costa Rica, the government is paying for all the medical services provided, so it has a strong incentive to prevent health problems before they happen. For every person in Costa Rica who doesn't get the flu or any other ailment, the government saves taxpayers money. That is one of the essential aspects of moving toward a single-payer government health care system. It transforms the system at the roots to make the government want to invest in prevention. Imagine if the government just spent the money needed to vaccinate the population against the flu instead of paying for the millions of dollars of hospital care required each flu season.

Our current system is set up to consider profits—of doctors, hospitals, insurance companies, and pharmaceutical companies—as a fundamental factor in determining how the system works. Imagine if we transformed our health care system to consider population health as the fundamental factor that determined how the system worked? That is essentially how Costa Rica's system works. The bottom line for them is health, not money. That is a huge shift from how we think about our health care system.

Ultimately, our country's capitalist values have been allowed to seep into our views about health care and how our health care system should operate. We think it is tragic but mundane for someone to go bankrupt because they had an illness. Imagine, though, if we viewed that as an unacceptable tragedy in our world? There may need to be difficult policy choices about health care provision because societal resources are limited, but the determination of who gets care should not be based on someone's bank account. Rather, there should be collective decisions about what is just and fair in the provision of health services.

If we take a prevention mindset, we will envision health care policies and a health care system that prioritizes preventing illnesses and accidents before they even begin. The system would be structured to incentivize prevention. Prevention would be built into the operations of health care providers and other societal systems. Success would be determined by how many illnesses and accidents are prevented rather than by how much profit is earned.

Medicare for All is an example of a policy approach that would be a huge step in this direction. It could transform the US health care system by giving the government more negotiating power—not just to decide how much to pay for different medical services and medicines but also to incentivize the type of care provided. For example, the government (e.g., the single payer) could require that any clinic or hospital providing services needs to ensure that transportation services are provided for patients, or that providers fund pipeline programs to diversify the medical workforce or have to undergo training on historical racism and its present-day impacts. The payer—aka the government, aka the taxpayer, aka the voters—would have tremendous power to shape the way that health care is delivered in this country.

People who accept the status quo will argue that policies like Medicare for All or other health care system changes are radical. But when you look at our system and the harms it has caused, what is actually radical? Is it radical to transform it or to spend trillions of dollars on pulling drowning people out of the river?

If we think about policies in line with a prevention mindset, we need to take the idea of Medicare for All even further by incorporating prevention into the health system overall, in the manner that Costa Rica has. According to the Centers for Disease Control, the United States spends $3.8 trillion on health care expenditures. Of that, only 2.6% is spent on public health and prevention activities.[61] In other words, 97.4% of our enormous health spending goes toward pulling drowning people from the river, and only a tiny sliver is spent on anything that might prevent the problem.

* * *

Health care is one of the most obvious areas where the policies we choose are about life and death. The current US system is not producing the health outcomes that peer countries are enjoying. Frankly, it is producing more deaths than it should, given how much US taxpayer money goes to it. To get the life and health benefits we deserve, we need to use our imagination, envision a different system, and work toward integrating a prevention mindset to transform the system at the roots.

Next, we will examine whether this same perspective can help us see new possibilities for our approach to environmental stewardship.

CHAPTER 4

Better Environment

Can We Thrive in a Burning World?

In the middle of July 1995, I had a baseball tournament in Mt. Prospect, about 20 miles northwest of Chicago. I remember hopping into my mom's turquoise-blue Dodge Caravan with my dusty bag of gear and driving 30 minutes north to get there.

My mom's minivan had a temperature reading in it just where the windshield met the car's roof. Like a lot of detail-oriented kids, I loved to know exactly what the precise temperature was. Before our minivan, our family's 1980s-era brown station wagon did not have the newfangled temperature technology. I would sit in the *wayback* and look out the window, scoping out display signs outside banks or strip malls that would display the temperature. But in the minivan, I could track it every time. The temperature reading that evening on the way to the tournament: 101 degrees Fahrenheit.

I remember playing that evening baseball game under the lights. I was out in left field, my hat brim soaked with sweat. The sun had gone down by then, but the temperature was still in the nineties. That heat was combined with a humidity that felt like someone was breathing on you. Parents brought coolers of ice with Gatorade in them to drink between innings. When we were on the bench, they had icy-cold towels to drape on our hot necks. The heat was stifling, but we had what we needed to manage.

I don't remember if we won or lost that game decades ago. But I do remember the feeling of that heat. It wasn't the last time I would feel temperatures that high, but it was the first time I have a vivid memory of it. After the game, I no doubt grabbed an icy-cold *pop* from some parent's cooler, guzzled it down, hopped into my parent's air-conditioned minivan, and arrived home to an air-conditioned house and a nice cool shower. It was steamy outside, but my family and I had a cool sanctuary that night.

Tragically, that wasn't true for many down the road in the city of Chicago. In what would become known as the 1995 Chicago heat wave, 485 people died in the city because of the heat in the two days before and after my sweaty Friday baseball game.[62] Though the heat wave hit several Midwestern states, including Iowa and Wisconsin, the deaths were concentrated in Chicago.

A combination of factors led to those deaths, but most scientists point to the "urban heat islands" in Chicago as a major contributing factor to the deaths. Some researchers showed that parts of the city that were primarily buildings and concrete were over 2 degrees Celsius hotter than other areas.[63] That is because concrete and traditional building materials absorb and retain heat rather than deflecting radiation from the sun. Areas of the city where poor Black residents lived were much less likely to have trees or green space that could better keep things cool. That was compounded by the fact that many poor residents did not have air conditioning or, if they did have it, were worried about the high electricity costs of turning it on. Some were even afraid to open their windows at night because of fear of being robbed.[64]

The local news that week focused on the number of people in Chicago who had died from the heat, many of them elderly. It was not a random cross-section of elderly Chicagoans. It was disproportionately Black and poor Chicagoans.[65] They were the people who were most likely to live in these urban heat islands and most likely to lack air conditioning or other supports. These deaths were tragic but ultimately preventable.

*   *   *

The Chicago heat wave was a climate disaster. In fact, it was one of the deadliest climate disasters in the United States, killing far more people than Superstorm Sandy did in 2012.[66]

But back in the 1990s, people were not talking about climate disasters the same way we recognize them now. Now, whenever we experience extreme weather, we know that there is a high likelihood that it is connected to our human-induced changing climate. In the summer of 2021, nearly one in three Americans experienced some sort of climate disaster (e.g., wildfires, floods, storms).[67]

As people know, Chicago isn't just really hot sometimes. It is also really cold sometimes. About seven months later, in the dead of winter, the temperatures dropped to –17 degrees Fahrenheit (–27 Celsius).[68] Thankfully, I did not have a baseball game that day, but I did take my black Labrador for a walk and tried to see if my spit would freeze before it hit the ground (it didn't). The Chicago area is built for that cold. We have heat, we have insulated pipes, we (mostly) have warming shelters for people who don't have shelter, and we (mostly) had a power grid that could handle the increased energy demand of heating. Texas isn't built that way.

Most of the United States watched a tragedy unfold when Texas experienced extreme weather in the middle of February 2021, with catastrophic results. The temperatures set records for being almost 50 degrees lower than average temps for that time of year. There were widespread power outages, flooding caused by pipes bursting, and people without shelter. In all, the Texas government determined that 246 people died, and it cost the Texas economy at least $80 billion.[69,70] While it seems counterintuitive, the extreme weather experienced in Texas was almost certainly due to human-caused global warming.[71]

The more carbon and other greenhouse gases that humans put into the atmosphere, the more our planet warms, which can cause extreme weather. The Arctic and Antarctic are warming faster than the rest of the planet, which can paradoxically cause cold weather extremes in other parts of the planet. The polar vortex is a band of low-pressure wind that keeps cold air trapped near the North Pole when the polar vortex is strong. But a warming planet has weakened the polar vortex. Climate researchers observed data and used predictive modeling to show that the warming Arctic is likely causing a disruption of the polar vortex that allows that cold air to dip further and further south into parts of the United States, including as far south as Texas.[72] So, while some skeptics like to point to unusual cold snaps as proof that climate change isn't serious, the opposite is actually true.

The Chicago heat wave and Texas cold snap will continue repeating themselves in the United States and across the world as temperatures creep up and extreme weather becomes more and more common. If our global emissions continue on the trajectory they are now, Chicago will likely see 30 days of 100-plus-degree heat in the future.[73] And of course, there are many other consequences to climate change other than just extreme weather events. We might see sea levels rise, wiping out certain countries and cities, as well as mass extinctions of certain species. In fact, we already are seeing such events.

Most people believe that human-induced climate change is a problem that emerged only recently, within the past three decades. But scientist and women's rights activist Eunice Foote conducted research in 1856 that showed that carbon dioxide was a greenhouse gas that could lead to global warming.[74] She concluded: "If the air had mixed with it a higher proportion of carbon dioxide than at present, an increased temperature" would occur.[75] When she conducted this research, the Earth had only about 285 parts per million (ppm) of carbon dioxide in the atmosphere compared to over 400 ppm today.[76] Human societies were just beginning to ramp up their burning of fossil fuels and, as industrialization took hold, would see an explosion of carbon dioxide emissions in the decades after Foote's scientific findings.

In 1896 (when carbon dioxide was still at 295 ppm), Swedish scientist and Nobel laureate Svante Arrhenius calculated that if carbon dioxide levels would continue to rise, the Earth's temperature would dramatically rise.[77] The broader public learned about the link between burning fossil fuels and global warming in a *Popular Mechanics* article in 1912 titled "Remarkable Weather of 1911: The Effect of the Combustion of Coal on the Climate—What Scientists Predict for the Future." That article states: *"It has been found that if the air contained more carbon dioxide, which is the product of the combustion of coal or vegetable material, the temperature would be somewhat higher."*[78]

When the *Popular Mechanics* article was released, the United States was just beginning to experience a steady rise in carbon dioxide emissions from fossil fuels. The US released about 1.3 billion tons of carbon emissions in 1912.[79] While that amount is still notable and well above the zero emissions goal, in recent years, US carbon dioxide emissions have increased to about 5 billion tons per year. The climate change we are experiencing now is mainly the result of the massive amount of greenhouse gases released over the past century.

We had opportunities to intervene then, but we didn't. We as a society have opted for a profit-driven stance rather than a prevention mindset. There were plenty of warnings before things got out of hand. At a conference of petroleum executives in 1959, an invited speaker warned about sea-level rise and flooded cities by reminding the attendees that "whenever you burn conventional fuel, you create carbon dioxide . . . its presence in the atmosphere causes a greenhouse effect."[80]

In 1965, President Lyndon B. Johnson's Science Advisory Committee released a report on atmospheric carbon dioxide that concluded: "By the year 2000 the increase in atmospheric CO_2 will be close to 25%." The report noted that this change in CO_2 levels would "almost certainly" cause temperature changes.[81] This government report did indeed get attention. Oil executives even discussed the report at a conference of the American Petroleum Institute (API)—their largest lobbying group. Two years later, in 1967, the US Senate was holding hearings on two bills that would help cut CO_2 emissions by promoting the development of electric vehicles and other, cleaner engine alternatives. A representative from the API testified in front of the Senate and lobbied against the bill, stalling its passage.[82] And oil companies continued to push for profits for decades while knowing the damage that atmospheric carbon dioxide was causing the environment and the climate. These were people operating in a bad system—a system where profits were incentivized over the health of our people and our planet. And we created that system with our public policies.

*   *   *

These climate changes are caused by humans. Policies (or lack of policies) related to the environment shape human and institutional actions related to climate change. Beyond climate change, environmental-related policies have an impact on our health and well-being. Mari Copeny and the other residents of Flint, Michigan, are one prime example of how current weak environmental protection policies can fail us. But there are many other ways that policy choices in this arena have led directly to the loss of life.

The policy decision to take weak or no action on climate change has already cost lives. A 2021 US study estimated that

174,000 deaths over the previous 20 years have been caused by extreme temperatures caused by human-induced climate change.[83] Of course, stemming climate change requires coordinated multinational action from countries beyond the United States. But, US policymakers have made it impossible to take bold action by either dragging their feet or outright abandoning global efforts. For example, the US Senate never ratified the Kyoto climate accords, which were adopted in 1997 by an international coalition of countries to stem climate change. Years later, in 2015–2016, the Paris climate accords tried to continue the work with the US as a key participant. Ultimately, these accords have been weakened because of backtracking by the administration of President Donald Trump in his first and second terms.[84]

With the largest economy, the United States is the largest historical emitter of greenhouse gases.[85] Its policymakers had the opportunity to lead the world toward transformative climate policies, but they chose not to. As a result of these policy choices, climate change is worsening and leading to increased disasters, excessive heat, and diseases that cause death.

Beyond these grave global consequences, our environmental policies have often allowed corporations to pollute water and air in local communities. While the amount of environmental regulations have oscillated depending on the political climate, US public policies for decades have given corporations excessive power to lobby for minimal oversight. A research study of 20 industrialized countries shows that industrial pollution significantly increases the death rate because industrial pollution is known to cause respiratory, lung, and cardiovascular health issues.[86] Corporate profit and economic growth have driven policy decisions more than protection of human life and well-being.

* * *

In the late 1950s, Charles Gelman, a graduate student in public health at the University of Michigan, was focused on detecting pollution or toxins in the air. He developed an instrument while he was doing work with the US Public Health Service that could detect air pollution. Ironically, this innovator in pollution detection to protect the public's health ended up creating a large multinational company that is the source of harmful groundwater contamination in my own community.[87]

After Gelman created his air pollution detector for his work with the US Public Health Service, he soon found that other people wanted to buy it. So, like so many other start-up founders, Gelman started a company in his basement. Eventually, the Gelman Instrument Company grew, and in the early 1960s, he moved himself and his 41 employees into a facility on the western outskirts of Ann Arbor, Michigan.

The business quickly thrived and grew. Gelman discovered a huge market for his work because of growing pollution in the environment. He said: "With growth of the country, expansion of industry, and the number of automobiles—all adding to pollution—we're not keeping pace," adding that "the trend toward pollution is running faster than the solutions for control."[87] His company was poised to fill the gap in the market by detecting pollution.

The new facility underwent expansion several times as the company succeeded and sold devices for measuring and controlling air and water pollution. All of this success meant that the company was manufacturing products using various chemicals and needed to discharge wastewater as part of the manufacturing process. The company tried different methods of discharging the wastewater.[88] It sprayed it on nearby fields and stored it in man-made lagoons on-site to be treated and discharged. Gelman claimed at the time that the wastewater was nontoxic.

But, concerns started to be raised as early as 1969. The State Water Resources Commission gave its lowest rating to the company because the lagoons were deemed inadequate. Neighbors started to raise concerns about a nearby lake being contaminated as well. Yet nothing really happened over the next decade, except further corporate expansion. By the end of the 1970s, the company had changed its name to Gelman Sciences, recorded $35 million in sales, and further expanded its facilities.[87]

As so often happens, all that financial success came at a cost to the environment and human health. In 1984, a graduate student at the same School of Public Health where Gelman had been a student—just three short miles from Gelman Sciences—took a sample from the nearby Third Sister Lake and discovered the presence of excessive amounts of 1,4-Dioxane.[89] This chemical may cause cancer and damage to the liver or kidneys when ingested through water.

Gelman Sciences was using dioxane as a solvent in some of its manufacturing processes. Almost 1 million pounds of dioxane was used over the course of two decades of manufacturing at the plant. Most of that was discharged to nearby soil, surface water, or groundwater.

The Third Sister Lake was not exactly a swimming hole or drinking water source, but it was soon determined that it was seeping into neighbors drinking wells, the groundwater, and water that was connected to the Huron River. Ann Arbor draws its drinking water for its over 100,000 residents from the Huron River.

Here's the thing about this whole issue: it came down to public policies and their implementation. After the discovery of excessive dioxane, the state of Michigan sued Gelman Sciences to force it to engage in cleanup efforts. But the judge ruled *in favor of* Gelman Sciences in 1991. According to an article in the *Ann Arbor News* at the time, the judge determined that with the exception of two small unauthorized spills, "all of Gelman's releases of the solvent were performed *under state issued permits.*"[90] The state of Michigan gave permits to allow for chemicals to be discharged into our environment. The public policy apparatus of the state that is intended to protect natural resources created conditions that allowed for contamination.

Eventually, the state and the Environmental Protection Agency (EPA) were able to compel Gelman Sciences to pay for some of the cleanup efforts. As of 2023, the dioxane spill was about to be listed as an EPA Superfund site on the National Priorities List, which includes thousands of other contaminated locations across the country that have hazardous waste.[91] The story of Gelman Sciences is just one of many such stories where lax policies and regulations inadequately protected people and our planet.

Ann Arbor is a relatively wealthy, well-educated, and a majority white city. This type of pollution and hazardous waste exposure is possible in any US town and location. Ann Arbor is proof of that. But like most other aspects of our society, harm is not distributed equally among all populations. The harm caused by Superfund sites and other polluting disproportionately affects residents who are poor and people of color.

* * *

Our policy choices over the past decades have perpetrated what is called environmental racism. Robert D. Bullard, the "father of environmental justice," defines environmental racism as:

> Any policy, practice, or directive that differentially affects or disadvantages (whether intended or unintended) individuals, groups, or communities based on race or color. It also includes exclusionary and restrictive practices that limit participation by people of color in decision-making boards, commissions, and regulatory bodies. Environmental racism exists within local zoning boards as well as the U.S. Environmental Protection Agency.[92]

This means that industrial pollutants, highways, landfills, and other harms have disproportionately been located near communities of color.

For example, the 48217 zip code in Southwest Detroit has been called the community with the most pollution in Michigan because an interstate highway, an oil refinery, a coal-fired power plant, and steel manufacturing are all located within it. According to the 2021 census estimates, there are almost 7,000 people that live there: 73% identify as Black, and 21% identify as Hispanic. The median household income in this zip code is $37,917, and the median value of owner-occupied houses is $42,200 (about 20% of the value of homes in the larger Detroit metro area).[93] One lifelong resident, Theresa Landrum, shared her experience: "My neighbors and I have been breathing in benzene, sulfur chloride, and hydrogen sulfide for years, and the health effects are clear. I've seen neighbors in their 20s die of cancer. I lost my mother and my father to cancer. I am a survivor."[94] How did it end up that Theresa and all her neighbors had to live with such concentrated pollution?

Our economic system of largely unregulated capitalism requires "sacrifice zones," or locations where the harms can be concentrated, like the 48217 zip code.[95] As policies and decisions are made, communities with the least power end up as sacrifice zones with concentrated harms. In US society, due to our legacy of white supremacy and structural racism, communities of color are often those with the least power. Thus, oil refineries and power plants are placed in communities of color rather than in wealthier and predominantly white suburbs or city neighborhoods. It is no accident that the census shows that only 2% of residents in the 48217 zip code identify as white. Other examples of sacrifice zones in the United States are "Cancer Alley" in Louisiana and more than 1,000 other hotspots known to increase risk for cancer (as documented by ProPublica).[96]

Hop Hopkins has been working for decades to help lead transformative change related to the environment. Shortly after racial justice protests erupted following the murder of George Floyd in 2020, Hopkins wrote an article titled "Racism Is Killing the Planet." The world had renewed focus on examining how racism and white supremacy was harming Black people and other people of color. Hopkins took the opportunity to emphasize how the harms of racism were connected to another monumental harm to human health: climate change. Hopkins succinctly wrote: "You can't have climate change without sacrifice zones, and you can't have sacrifice zones without disposable people, and you can't have disposable people without racism."[97]

We as a country have allowed so much harm and contamination simply because the people with the most power (e.g., wealthy, white, and educated) have been able to minimize their own exposure to the harms. They don't live in Cancer Alley. They don't live next to the polluting factory. The captains of industry don't build their industry in their backyard.

Homeowners crying *not-in-my-backyard* is such a thing that it has a name: NIMBYism. And NIMBYism is one of the reasons that environmental racism is so rampant. Property owners with the most wealth and power in society are effectively able to organize and lobby to ensure that a new industrial site or highway with polluting cars is not built near their homes. Or, more often, they are sufficiently respected that their neighborhood is not even considered to begin with. They also often use this NIMBY power to prevent the construction of affordable housing or anything on the green space surrounding their home or neighborhood.[98]

People with less power in society have had less success fighting these harms because powerful interests who want to build a factory or highway are often better able to mobilize support from politicians and other decision-makers. But marginalized communities have a long history of fighting back, just like Mari

Copeny is doing in Flint. In zip code 48217, residents have been fighting against polluters for the health and well-being of their neighborhood for many decades. In Chicago, residents from the Southeast Side have long fought against pollutants being placed in their neighborhood. Recently, residents fought against General Iron moving into a predominantly Latino neighborhood by staging a hunger strike and various other forms of advocacy.[99] They were successful, but it took a years-long campaign. Have you ever heard of wealthy white home-owners staging a hunger strike? They have too many other cards to play to draw the attention of decision-makers. They can hire a lawyer to sue, they can threaten to withhold political donations, and they can get the news to cover their issue.

When disaster strikes, whether it is a heat wave in Chicago, a cold snap in Texas, or lead in the water in Michigan, it strikes most harshly within poor and racially marginalized communities. Our public policy choices are causing harm to our planet and its residents. While our country has outright avoided implementing environmental protection policies, even the measures that we have adopted have been insufficient to ward off harms. It is time to imagine and follow a different path.

Imagining a Better World: Policies Based on a Prevention Mindset

There are no simple fixes when it comes to climate change. In a speculative fiction novel by Kim Stanley Robinson called *The Ministry of the Future*, the author narrates the story of some of the climate-related tragedies that will occur in the coming decades and how the global community comes together to fight climate change.[100] Although it is ultimately a hopeful novel, there is certainly a lot of heartache. Namely, millions-dead-from-a-heat-wave type of heartache. Overwhelming-numbers-of-climate-refugees type of heartache. Collapsing-global-economic-systems type of heartache. I certainly hope that the future does not come to that, but it could if we do not take a different course with our public policies.

It is easy to think individual behavior change could be the solution. If we could all just compost, stop buying things we don't need, cut down on air travel, avoid eating animal products, buy an electric car, and live in a modest-size house, we would be doing our part to stop climate change. If we could get most people in society to follow the same advice, we would all be using so much less carbon and therefore reduce the release of greenhouse gases.

But, relying on individual behavior change—especially without any support or positive consequences—is an uphill battle. As an example, consider that when COVID vaccines were made available, some portion of the population immediately went out to receive them simply based on the recommendation and evidence provided by experts. But then there were two other segments of the population: (1) those who did not believe or trust expert advice and (2) those who could not take off work, find transportation, or otherwise had barriers to getting a timely vaccine. We see similar groups when thinking about climate-related behavior change. Relying on individual choices will be too slow. We need to reorient our society to consider people and the planet before profits.

The concepts behind the Green New Deal offer one vision for a path forward. The Green New Deal has been an idea that has been discussed over the past two decades, but it came to greater prominence when US Representative Alexandria Ocasio-Cortez and Senator Ed Markey introduced legislation to the US Congress in 2018.[101]

The Green New Deal legislation in the United States is intentionally expansive. Predictably, this ambitious legislation includes elements specific to the environment like "smart power grid" or "removing pollution and greenhouse gas emissions from the transportation and agricultural sectors." It also includes provisions that are less directly related to the environment like "millions of high-wage union jobs" and "providing higher education, high-quality health care, and affordable, safe, and adequate housing to all." The rationale behind including both is a recognition that individuals who have to make their political and consumption decisions from a place of fear—fear of an economy leaving behind people without a bachelor's degree, fear of a medical bankruptcy, or fear of eviction or foreclosure—are unable to prioritize the health of the planet. To create an economy and society where both the people and the planet have what they need to thrive, proponents of the Green New Deal advocate for an economy with a strong social safety net, worker rights, and attention to redressing historical harms for marginalized communities.

Promotion of equity and justice for historically marginalized communities is one of the key goals of the Green New Deal, and it is incorporated throughout the proposed legislation. It is clear that those marginalized groups—the legislation lists "indigenous peoples, communities of color, migrant communities, deindustrialized communities, depopulated rural communities, the poor, low-income workers, women, the elderly, the unhoused, people with disabilities, and youth"—are often hit hardest by a changing climate and changing economy and by the current harms of our existing economy.[101]

To make sure resources and protections flow into these communities, one key measure within the legislation is "ensuring the use of democratic and participatory processes that are inclusive of and led by frontline and vulnerable communities and workers."[101] If implemented, this would mean that the groups listed above would be at the center of decision-making processes about green investments and environmental regulations. This has the potential to eliminate the sacrifice zones that have pro-liferated under our current economic system. By prioritizing communities of people instead of economic profit and corpora-tions, this legislation can create a society that minimizes harm to people and the planet.

While the Green New Deal would be a huge step forward in addressing environmental injustice and climate change, some argue it does not go far enough. The Green Party in the United States, which helped to originate the ideas behind the Green New Deal before the Democrats in Congress adopted it, is more detailed and specific in its proposal about the ways that the capi-talist economy needs to be upended to put these proposals into action.[102]

Others are also pushing for a more transformative vision of society to address climate change and create a more sustainable society. The Red Nation—a US-based Native American advocacy group focused on the liberation of Indigenous peoples—released the Red Deal in 2021 as an extension of the Green New Deal.[103] The Red Deal calls for a return of land to Indigenous peoples and ways of being. Our current planetary crisis is framed as a prob-lem where the root cause is capitalism and colonization and the solution is returning to Indigenous forms of land stewardship and governance—specifically, minimizing hierarchy in society and treating "nonhuman relatives" like the land, water, and an-imals with true care and respect.

Other Indigenous leaders have emphasized that one of the root causes of our planetary crisis is the broader culture's will-ingness to separate humans from the rest of nature. Is it this mental distortion—claiming that humans are not part of nature and are not connected to it—that allows people and their public policies to treat the planet as a resource to be exploited rather than respected. Enrolled member of the Citizen Potawatomi Na-tion and decorated professor Robin Kimmerer describes how the

Potawatomi language refers to humans similarly to other objects and beings in nature. They are all alive, not an "it," but rather an animate being. In her book *Braiding Sweetgrass*, she writes:

> Our toddlers speak of plants and animals as if they were people, extending to them self and intention and compassion—until we teach them not to. We quickly retrain them and make them forget. When we tell them that the tree is not a who, but an it, we make that maple an object; we put a barrier between us, absolving ourselves of moral responsibility and opening the door to exploitation.[104]

This "barrier between us" that Kimmerer describes gives us all license to harm in different ways and to merely focus on the benefit of humans. But, to truly transform our society and get to the root cause of the problems, we need to fundamentally shift how we think about our relationship to the Earth. Enrique Salmón is from the Rarámuri (Tarahumara) tribe of northwestern Mexico and an ethnobotanist who coined the term *kincentric* ecology. He wrote:

> Indigenous people view both themselves and nature as part of an extended ecological family that share ancestry and origins. It is an awareness that life in any environment is viable only when humans view the life surrounding them as kin. The kin, or relatives, include all the natural elements of an ecosystem. Indigenous people are affected by and, in turn, affect the life around them. The interactions that result from this "kincentric ecology" enhance and preserve the ecosystem.[105]

If we can move more toward this idea of kincentric ecology, in both our public policies and voters attitudes, we can work toward creating a sustainable future.

The Green New Deal and other policy proposals to shift our public policies to become more sustainable and equitable are important steps to take in the (hopefully) short term if we want to stem climate change and redress the environmental harms experienced by mostly marginalized communities. But, in the longer term, we need to take a critical lens to how our culture thinks about its relationship with the Earth.

CHAPTER 5

Better Education

Are Schools a Ladder or a Sieve?

When I started my job as a faculty member, they assigned me to serve on an admissions committee. I had applied to colleges once and graduate schools twice—and had helped several family members and friends in their own personal essays and applications—and now I was going to be someone that read and evaluated those applications to decide whether someone would be eligible to enroll in our degree program.

I am someone who wonders about the life story of every stranger or acquaintance I encounter. Where are they from? What do they do? What are they interested in? What are their goals? I am a people person and curious about the people around me. So, the work of reviewing applicant essays and transcripts and recommendation letters definitely had elements that were interesting and fun. We were admitting graduate students to our public health school, and many of the applicants had deeply compelling experiences that pushed them into our field (some were also deeply boring).

Starting in December, our administrator would start to pass along admissions files. I had to remember my password, log on to the system, and see the list of applicants I was responsible for reviewing and scoring. Each one had a pdf file I could download that contained their answers to the numerous questions they were asked as part of the application process, their personal essays, their transcript, and three recommendation letters. There was a lot of biography and background to sift through!

My job was ultimately to decide if I thought that an applicant could succeed in the program. Our philosophy as a department was to view applicants holistically; a GPA or a test score or some other "negative" aspect could not completely hold a candidate back. We gave second chances, and we knew that not everyone excels in everything. Mostly, we were looking to weed out applicants whose interests and goals were a mismatch for what our program could offer and those who might struggle academically and require a level of support that we simply could not provide.

I had a problem, though. I wanted to accept almost everyone. I felt—and feel—like our field is amazing, and everyone would benefit from our program. If they wanted to come study in our program, my heart wanted to let them. I struggled with my role as gatekeeper.

The other aspect that I struggled with was the incredibly phenomenal applicants who would end up rejecting our offer of admission because of how expensive it was. While we do give out many scholarships, oftentimes they are not for full tuition. A scholarship may only be for a quarter or half the cost of tuition. And many people who are admitted receive no scholarships. In 2024, the cost to attend our program was almost $18,000 per semester if you are lucky enough to live in Michigan. As a state university, we charged people from outside Michigan over $29,000 *per semester* to attend. As a full-time residential program, most students need to move to Ann Arbor and can only manage to do small part-time jobs for the duration of their two-year (four semester) program. When you consider all of this together, my university's office of financial aid estimates a student from Michigan will need over $64,000 to cover expenses for one academic year (not including the summer period), and a student from outside Michigan will need over $87,000 for each of the two years of the program.[106] To complete our two-year program without any scholarships, students will need to spend well over $100,000 and in some cases much more. A degree in my field definitely has the potential to boost earnings, but the cost-benefit financially is not necessarily a slam dunk.

Some of our applicants simply cannot make it work; they cannot take two years off from earning money, and they cannot take out massive loans. They may already be saddled with undergraduate debt, and they do not have the confidence that the world they live in will reward them enough for a graduate degree to make it worth it. Or they simply need to prioritize the basic needs of loved ones rather than invest those resources in an expensive degree program. And those students who do take the plunge and take out tens of thousands (if not hundreds of thousands) of dollars in loans can be in a difficult situation trying to pay them back.

So, as I sat reviewing the detailed information about every internship, every passion, and every goal, I could not help but wonder what system I was contributing to. It is my profession to provide higher education. But, by creating such an expensive product, are we withholding this product from people who are not advantaged enough to be able to pay for it?

We often like to think of education as a ladder extended to students from any background to give them a boost to climb to a better future. But sociology researchers summarizing the research on higher education have noted that "formal education has been less of a ladder than a social sieve, regulating access to privileged social positions."[107]

We use education and degree programs, in part, to decide who gets to do what in society. A bachelor's degree is increasingly required for access to the middle class, despite its astronomical cost. In my field of public health, an MPH degree is typically required for most management or leadership positions. We rarely discuss it in such stark terms, but we are essentially saying that people have to pay tens of thousands of dollars for the opportunity to be a manager or to be in the middle class. For people who are from the middle or upper classes, their families may be able to provide enough support or stability to make that possible. But for those with limited resources, they can hope for scholarships or take on a massive student-loan burden with the hope that it will pay off. And scholarships and loans are only helpful if you have made it all the way to the collegiate or graduate level. What about the students at the K–12 level who do not receive enough support to even know how to go about creating a competitive application? Do we not want those people to be working in fields like public health, law, or medicine that usually demand high education and college or graduate degrees? Is that the choice we want to be making as a society?

* * *

Our education policies, including costs related to education, can shape who lives, who dies, and who thrives in our society. I am a proud product of public schools. I went to public schools from kindergarten through grade 12. My education continued at the publicly funded University of Illinois for my undergraduate degree and the publicly funded University of North Carolina for my doctorate. I currently work at the publicly funded University of Michigan.

My own K–12 public school experience was adequately funded and set me up for success. My teachers were unionized and some of the best-paid public schoolteachers in the state of Illinois. Our buildings and facilities were safe and well maintained, our classrooms were not overcrowded, and we had the textbooks and materials needed to learn. My parents had the financial ability to choose our town specifically because of the high-quality public schools. This excellent K–12 education set me up for a successful college application to our state's flagship university, which then helped set me up for graduate school and a successful career. During my K–12 education, there were plenty of resources available to families like mine because of public policies that allowed certain districts to have more resources than others.

Funding for schools draw primarily from property taxes within individual districts, and state or federal funding tries to fill in the gap. But some students with greater needs are often left underresourced. The district that I lived in was relatively wealthy, so the public schools were well-funded and had a low proportion of high-need students. Students who lived in school districts in poorer areas of the state did not have all the same advantages that I did. And these advantages—or disadvantages—translate into people's health and well-being.

Well-funded high-quality schools can keep kids in school and improve their educational attainment. Educational attainment has been causally linked to health in the United States. People who are college educated enjoy the best health while those who have only a high school degree or less have the worst health. Some evidence suggests that for every two additional years of schooling, you can expect to live an extra year of life.[108] This is largely due to the fact that college graduates in white-collar jobs usually receive higher wages and better health insurance, which sometimes are not available to people in other types of jobs with lower levels of education. There is so much beyond a student's control—and shaped by policy—that determines whether they continue their schooling. And yet, life chances are often shaped by how many years of schooling you have.

In the United States, there are massive inequities in what type of education is possible depending on your zip code, how much money your parents have, or what your racial identity is. Whether a student chooses to graduate high school or attend college is not merely an individual choice—it is strongly influenced by the policy environment and the resources accessible to the student. If you live in New York State, your state government's budgetary policy spends about $23,000 per student. If you live in Oklahoma, your policymakers have only allocated about $8,000 per student.[109] How much support you have to continue schooling has a lot to do with state, local, and school-level policies.

Our systems of higher education are no better. Rather than public policies at the state or federal level that create a university system that keeps barriers to education low, we have a system where the very best universities—both private and public—charge exorbitant tuition. Even state schools, like the one where I work, still charge an incredible amount of money for a degree. In today's dollars, a student at a public university in 1970 could expect to pay about $2,500 per year for tuition and fees. Fifty years later, the cost is more than three times higher, costing a student $9,349 per year on average to attend a *government-subsidized* public school.[110] Private schools are even more expensive, costing $32,769 per year on average. Of all OECD countries, the United States has among the highest tuition (Canada and Australia cost about half as much), and several OECD countries charge $0 for college tuition.[111]

At the state and federal level, public funding for higher education has decreased substantially over the past several decades. Students now pay almost 50% of all educational costs in tuition, compared to only about 25% in 1988.[112] This prohibitive cost of education prevents people from obtaining the enhanced health outcomes associated with more education. Further, it created an incredible amount of student debt that is linked to poor mental and physical health among borrowers.[113]

State policies can offer free or substantially discounted college tuition for low-income students to help them continue their education beyond high school. For example, the University of Michigan has implemented the "Go Blue Guarantee," which, as of fall 2025, provides free tuition for college students whose families earn less than $125,000 per year and have less than $125,000 in assets. Many other colleges and universities have similar policies; while it is a step in the right direction, it does not solve all the college affordability problems.

There are other types of policies, beyond funding, that can affect a student's life trajectory and opportunities. Policies related to discipline and policing within schools create very different situations for students depending on their zip code or racial identity. Black and Latino students are disproportionately subject to school-to-prison pipeline policies that expel them from high schools for minor infractions, refer them to police, and ultimately place them in jails or prisons.[114] Policies related to what the curriculum is, how teachers are trained, and what social services are provided within schools also can have an important effect on what types of students thrive and are able to succeed in school compared to those who do not.[115]

Providing a good education is a big part of thinking about prevention policies. When we deprive a segment of our population of a good education and opportunities early in life, it can have downstream effects on society. If someone is deprived of the opportunity for high-quality education and a pathway to a middle-class job, it can mean they are trapped in poverty, lack health insurance coverage, and suffer the negative health consequences of that combination. Public policies that provide strong educational opportunities for everyone within society are a vital component of implementing prevention policies.

Imagining a Better World: Policies Based on a Prevention Mindset

Let us start with our goals for an education system. What outcomes do we want? We likely want all young people to be able to develop critical skills to function and thrive in society. If we care at all about equity, we want *all* young people to have the opportunities and resources they need to succeed in this system. We also want to have a population that has the skills to fill the jobs in our society.

If we use the prevention mindset, what is it that we want to prevent? We want to prevent the waste of human resources through differential access to opportunities. So, if we start from scratch, what do we need in our education system?

Finland provides an interesting example of a different model of public education. Chris Weller writes in *The Independent* about eight reasons that Finland's education system puts the US system to shame:

1. Competition isn't as important as cooperation.
2. Teaching is one of the most respected professions.
3. Finland listens to the research.
4. Finland is not afraid to experiment.
5. Playtime is sacred.
6. Kids have very little homework.
7. Preschool is high-quality and universal.
8. College tuition is free.[116]

Just looking at this list, we can see some fundamental differences between US schools and Finland's system. Not all of these reasons will necessarily be the right fit for our country, but it helps remind us that our system—defined by low-paid teachers, limited universal preschool, a lot of competition, and unequal funding—is a choice and that alternatives do exist.

*   *   *

One policy transformation that has received increased attention is free college tuition for all. This policy proposal fundamentally shifts the dynamics of our higher education system from one that is a commodity to one that is a public good. Given the ways that an educated populace benefits society and the economy, this public investment in higher education makes good sense.

What are the proposals and the evidence? In the United States, Senator Bernie Sanders's proposal of free college tuition for all is perhaps most well-known. During his presidential campaign, he proposed eliminating tuition and fees at all four-year public colleges and universities, tribal colleges, community colleges, trade schools, and apprenticeship programs. This is currently how many countries across the globe, including Germany, Norway, Kenya, and others, treat their higher education system.

In 2023, the College for All Act was introduced in the US Congress by Senator Bernie Sanders from Vermont and US Representative Pramila Jayapal from Washington. This legislation proposed to make all community colleges tuition- and fee-free for all students; public four-year colleges and historically Black colleges and universities (HBCUs) and minority-serving institutions would be tuition-free and fee-free for single households earning less than \$125,000/year and married households earning less than \$250,000 per year.[117] The proposal would guarantee that the federal government takes on 80% of the cost, with states and territories taking on the rest of the costs.

This bill, and other proposals to make education more accessible and affordable, view education—including higher education—as a public good rather than a commodity. Since higher education is a pathway to the middle class and better health within our society, it is critical to remove the barriers to this public good. But college comes toward the end of formal schooling, so we need to think about public policies that can promote equity in the earlier stages of formal education.

* * *

Study after study shows that kindergarten is too late to start a public education system.[118] By the time kids reach kindergarten, there are big differences in preparation that often last throughout someone's school trajectory. Research shows that investing in preschoolers helps prevent poor outcomes later in life and helps those children and their families thrive.

Head Start is a federally funded school readiness program focused on low-income kids ages 0–5 that was originally created by President Lyndon B. Johnson as part of his Great Society domestic policies. Currently, Head Start preschools provide free or low-cost education for kids between the ages of 3 and 5. These programs have been extensively studied and show that the investment early in life pays dividends later in life.[119]

One study by the National Institute for Early Education Research at Rutgers University found that high-quality universal preschool would close the achievement gap for reading at kindergarten entry between white students and Black or Latino students.[120] It also would narrow the gap between low-income and higher-income students.

Even early preschool programs cannot fix everything. For kids to have equal opportunities, we will have to fix inequities that their parents experience and, of course, fix the educational systems that they will enter into for kindergarten and beyond. But the investment in early childhood education—at a critically sensitive time in a child's life—is aligned with an upstream and prevention mindset for education policy.

*   *   *

One of the other root causes of an unequal education system is our current funding model. According to the Peter G. Peterson Foundation, nearly 40% of funding for public education stems from local property taxes.[121] Wealthier locales are able to fund their schools at a high level. States also provide funding and typically attempt to overcome some of the inequities caused by the local property tax model by providing more money to less wealthy districts. They also usually have formulas that allocate funds based on how many students are under the poverty line, how many are English-language learners, and other markers of disadvantage. But, ultimately, this finance model does not overcome the inequities throughout the system.

If we are guided by principles of equity (rather than just equality), our public policies should be allocating resources based on need. Districts with the most students living in poverty or from marginalized groups should receive the most funding to help them overcome those systematic disadvantages. While some state funding models do try to take this equity approach, too often marginalized communities do not have the resources they need to help students thrive.

Often, districts with high poverty are wrestling with providing numerous resources for their students who are coming to school with more complex issues because of the circumstances of their poverty or marginalization. They simply need more resources to help their students overcome the numerous barriers to their success.

More resources do not always immediately lead to better outcomes. When chronically underfunded districts get an increase in funding, sometimes all they can do is spend it on overdue repairs or other things that do not immediately translate into better learning outcomes. But there is evidence that when poorer districts advocate for more funding and receive it, the students in those districts benefit. One nationally representative study by the National Bureau of Economic Research found that low-income students who were in a district where school spending increased steadily throughout their schooling years were more likely to graduate high school, less likely to be poor as adults, and experienced an almost 10% increase in their adult income.[122]

More money for poor school districts is necessary but insufficient to truly give all students equal opportunity to learn and thrive. The experience of school districts trying to support their poor and marginalized students with the most need makes a strong case for strengthening our social safety net for all communities. This would ensure that the families of these students have access to health care, safe and affordable housing, basic income, and sustenance. Beyond a social safety net, these families also need to have the same chances to flourish as their counterparts in wealthier communities, without facing surveillance and criminalization. Part of addressing the school funding issues is to invest in marginalized communities and work toward reducing inequities overall in society.[123,124]

* * *

Beyond funding, we can think about education policies helping to create schools as community hubs. Around the country, we see that schools have sports fields, playgrounds, and sometimes community gardens that can be used by their surrounding communities. But what if we connected other vital resources into a school community?

Some states and districts are experimenting with school-based health centers that put doctors, nurses, and other health care professionals directly within schools to provide immunizations, well-child visits, mental health services, chronic disease management (e.g., asthma, diabetes), and other vital health care services for young people. These types of services remove a vital barrier to care for youth, especially poor or other disadvantaged youth, by integrating health care into their daily school life. There is strong evidence that school-based health centers can increase access to care, improve health outcomes, enhance school achievement, and ensure better uptake of important vaccinations.[125,126] Some of these school-based health centers also extend health services for students' families or younger siblings, helping to fill a gap and offering convenience within communities.

These school-based health centers align with the concept of "community schools." Community schools, which differ from neighborhood schools, encourage a closer relationship between schools and their surrounding communities, linking instruction and engaging in co-planning to ensure that the school is meeting the community's needs.[127] In this vein, we can start to think of schools as hubs of resources where community members are frequently interfacing with their neighbors and being connected to needed resources. A study of a school district in Albuquerque found that simply hiring a community school coordinator to help build those connections between school and community led to a $7 return on every dollar invested in the salary of the coordinator.[128]

As our communities and neighborhoods have become increasingly disconnected over the decades—famously documented in the book *Bowling Alone* by Robert Putnam[129]—community schools could start to increase connections and fill gaps within communities. To do this effectively, schools would need additional resources and staff; it should not be done at the expense of existing school budgets.

What would it look like if families could enroll in SNAP (Supplemental Nutrition Assistance Program) and Medicaid after they drop their kids off at school? What if they could get connected to job training and employment resources after they check-in with their child's teacher? What if immigration legal services and language classes were readily available with child-care provided? Certainly, some districts and school social workers already provide some of these services, but a truly transformed idea of what a school is to a community could create opportunities for integrated and interconnected resources within a community.

* * *

Ultimately, our education system must undergo many other transformations to ensure that all people can thrive. Curriculum, teacher training, and community support are all relevant factors. But much of it comes down to the budget and the resources we are willing to invest in education and training. Whether its college, K–12, or preschool, our current investments are inequitably distributed and are a root cause of inequities across society. By adopting a prevention mindset, we can position our education system to prevent inequities instead of worsening them.

CHAPTER 6

Better Justice

Are Prisons a Good Investment?

My cousin Paul was much older than me. Actually, he was only about a decade younger than my dad. I always had an affinity for my cousin because we shared the same name, and as a kid, I thought that was so cool. But, as a kid, I mostly only knew Paul through stories; he was in prison for most of my childhood.

Paul's childhood was more challenging than mine. He grew up in Detroit during a tumultuous time for the city, and he was a middle child of six kids. He had a goofy sense of humor and an easygoing personality. But he ended up spending much of his adult life in prison.

I was lucky enough to have never visited a jail or prison before. As a young kid, like a lot of other kids, I played "cops and robbers" with my friends. In the game, hiding under the bed, behind the couch, or in a closet was a pretend jail. Enemies and bad people were sent to prison, simple as that. Even today, I hear my son trying to put his younger sisters in jail when they are playing. Jail is apparently an appealing idea for anyone who is not behaving exactly how you would like them to.

But despite my pretend play, being imprisoned was still a fairly abstract concept to me as a kid since my community had not been targeted by the mass incarceration and war on drugs policies of the 1980s. The fact that I had an incarcerated cousin was a bit of a novelty to my mostly white suburban friends. As far as

I knew, none of them had any family members in prison. This contrasts with many people who are part of marginalized communities. For example, 63% of Black Americans have had a close family member incarcerated.

When I was about eight, my dad offered to bring me along on a visit to Paul, who was imprisoned in another state. After we passed through metal detectors and registered with uniformed guards, we entered a visiting area—a nondescript room with round tables—where we were able to sit and talk with my cousin. Paul was friendly and joked around with my dad and me; he was grateful to have us make the effort to visit.

I would see Paul again a few years later at a family reunion after he was released. He was as goofy as ever, and it was fun to see him again in a more casual environment. But he would do another stint in prison shortly thereafter. When he got out again, we went to a Chicago Cubs baseball game. We were both excited about the opportunity to connect now that I was a young adult. Unfortunately, he got drawn back in for a third stint in prison shortly after that.

He was released for the last time when he was well into middle age. The years on the inside had taken their toll on him. His similar-aged siblings were doing well, but Paul was struggling with health issues and looked older than his age. He made a go at life on the outside and reconnected with family members. But, tragically, he passed away in 2021 at the age of 55 from chronic illnesses, 20 years earlier than the life expectancy for white men in this country.

I would later learn from public health research that for every year of incarceration, a person is estimated to lose two years of life.[130] So, if someone spends 10 years in prison, on average they die 20 years earlier than would otherwise be expected. Paul's premature death at age 55 was about what the research predicted. Prison simply is not an environment that promotes good physical and mental health. In terms of lost life expectancy, spending six years in prison is on par with getting lung cancer.[131]

As a kid, I thought jails and prisons were a natural part of any society. Someone is bad or breaks the law, they get put in prison. Prison abolitionists dream of and try to build a world where there are no prisons. Some might wonder, if we did not have prisons, where would we put all the people who break the law? But this perspective diminishes the humanity of people like my cousin Paul. People who have made a mistake or caused harm to society do not necessarily need to be "put somewhere." As Angela Davis has said, "prisons do not disappear problems, they disappear human beings."[132]

Our public policies in this arena are aiming to address social harms like theft and violence. But our system of prisons and other criminal legal policies are not necessarily addressing the root cause of these issues. A prison sentence—or even parole or probation—does not usually rehabilitate. Even worse, it can cause harm to individuals and communities. So should we invest this much money in prisons—about $80 billion annually—and what alternatives could we envision?

* * *

Criminal legal policies are intended to maintain public safety and respond to the societal problems of violence, theft, and other harms. Our criminal legal system typically metes out consequences in the form of fines, prison, or probation in an effort to deter people from engaging in activities deemed criminal and to punish (and possibly rehabilitate) people who commit criminal activities. This deterrence, punishment, and rehabilitation strategy will supposedly reduce the harms that occur in a given community. Research indicates, however, that there is little evidence that our current punitive legal system actually prevents these harms.

From 1993 to 2022, the rate of reported violent victimization (e.g., rape or sexual assault, robbery, aggravated assault, and simple assault) dropped from 80 reported crimes per 1,000 people to 24 per 1,000 people.[133] These dramatic drops are mirrored in statistics on reported murder rates and property crimes.[134] While there was a slight increase in crimes reported to police in the early 2020s, the rate is still drastically lower than it was three decades ago. If we look at that same period of 1993 to 2022, the rate of incarceration in the United States increased from about 5.3 per 1,000 people in 1993 to 6.4 per 1,000 people in 2019.[135] Did this increase in the prison rate help reduce crime?

A report by the Vera Institute of Justice documented that the drop in crime rates in the first two decades of the 2000s had nothing to do with the rise in incarceration during that period.[136] It had more to do with an aging population, increased wages, increased employment, and increased graduation rates.

There is little evidence that incarceration plays a deterrent effect, either. A study of people who committed violent crimes showed that prison is no more effective than probation at deterring someone from committing a future violent crime.[137] Crafting public policy to prevent the harms of violence or theft and promote public safety is crucial for any society, yet the public policy solution of incarceration does not have a strong evidence base to support it.

Criminal legal policies have an expansive impact on people's lives. First, we know that the criminal legal system directly takes lives by executing about 20 people each year and keeping 200,000 people fully captive with life sentences.[138,139] These policy choices are harming people and communities in very direct ways, but the life-or-death consequences of our criminal legal system extend beyond those who are incarcerated to their family members and communities.

A rigorous analysis of nationally representative and longitudinal data showed that young adults whose father has been incarcerated are more likely to be diagnosed with high cholesterol, asthma, migraine, depression, posttraumatic stress disorder, and anxiety than young adults without an incarcerated father (even after controlling for sociodemographic factors and characteristics of the family).[140] The impact on health has even been shown to extend beyond a direct connection within one's family. There is evidence that people living in neighborhoods with a high percentage of people going to prison are about twice as likely to be depressed or have anxiety, regardless of neighborhood income, violent crime rates, and racial makeup.[141] The societal investment in prisons does not just cause poor health for those who are incarcerated, it has spillover effects into the well-being of families and communities.

*   *   *

Beyond the general harms that incarceration policies can have, they also have disproportionate impact on some groups of people. There is a concept called "discretion" within the criminal legal system that injects a lot of bias into the system and creates vast inequities.[142] Discretion used by prosecutors, judges, and parole officers at every step of the criminal legal system determines what types of laws get prosecuted, who gets bail, who gets maximum sentences, and who gets parole. Just like elsewhere in our society, discrimination and biases based on race, gender, and wealth shape these decisions.[143,144] Proximity to wealth, power, and whiteness protects people from arrest, prosecution, and prison. The people prosecuted and jailed for drug possession, for example, are not usually the white college students smoking pot in their dorm or the Wall Street bankers who snort cocaine.

At a societal level, this discretion means that we put people in prison only for certain types of harms, like burglary or violence, but not others, like corporate pollution, manipulating the financial system, or wage theft by employers. The 2008 financial crisis caused harm to millions of people because bankers illegally manipulated the mortgage market for their own gain. Despite the harm caused, none of the executives or bankers who created the toxic mortgage products was arrested or jailed.[145] Compare that to Wayne Bryant, a Black man who was sentenced to life in prison in Louisiana for attempting to steal a pair of hedge clippers.[146]

Because of the discretion built across the system, the deaths and other harm caused by the criminal legal system are not randomly distributed across the population. Instead, they disproportionately affect Black, Latino, and Native American residents, people who are homeless or experience mental health issues, and people who are sexual or gender minorities. Further, we have often criminalized mental illness that can manifest as a "public nuisance" or "disorderly conduct" and homelessness, which manifests as "loitering." It is thus unsurprising that almost half of all prisoners have a mental health disorder.[147]

Despite the known harms (and likely *because* the harms of our current system rarely touch upper-class white people), the United States has invested heavily in policies that incarcerate people, especially poor and racially marginalized residents. We have the highest incarceration rate in the world, imprisoning about 7 of every 1,000 residents compared to only 1 out of every 1,000 residents for Europe or Canada. This amounts to over 2 million people held in captivity at an estimated cost of $42,672 per person per year in 2022.[148] Given that the 2022 median personal annual income in the United States was $40,480, we are choosing public policies that use tax dollars to pay more than an annual wage to punish someone in a way that will prevent them from working productively, caring for their loved ones, or contributing to their community.[149] And, ultimately, research shows that these policies reduce their life expectancy and decrease the health of their families and communities.

The amount of our taxes that we put toward incarcerating people is a policy decision. A report by the Institute for Justice Research and Development at Florida State University showed that over $80 billion per year in taxpayer money was spent on incarceration.[150] By comparison, the Environmental Protection Agency—tasked with the mission to "protect human health and the environment"—had a fiscal year (FY) 2022 annual budget of $9.6 billion.[151] The highly effective Special Supplemental Nutrition Program for Women, Infant, and Children (WIC) had a FY2023 budget of $5.7 billion to provide services for 6.3 million individuals *per month*.[152]

Beyond the actual costs of incarcerating, there are costs to the communities and families where incarcerated people are from. The report by the Institute for Justice Research and Development showed that for every dollar spent by the state on incarcerating someone, there is an additional $10 of "social costs." An estimated $500 billion is born directly by the families, children, and communities of incarcerated individuals.[150]

Imagining a Better World: Policies Based on a Prevention Mindset

Chicago-based artist Olly Costello created a piece of art that shows the silhouettes of three people flying amidst the night sky while intermingled with starry constellations. Above them are the words: "If we have the imagination for mass incarceration then we have the imagination for mass freedom." It is hard to think that if we were creating a society from scratch that we would want to spend $80 billion to keep 1.9 million of our residents in jails or prisons.[153]

What would you do if your beloved brother stole $100 from your purse? Would you call the police and try to get him criminally tried? Would you want him to be punished with jail time? In Michigan, where I live, stealing $100 is punishable by up to 93 days in jail. Is that what you would want for your loved one?

Part of the issue with our current incarceration system is that we do not envision people who have committed harms as deserving of care and support. As a society, we call them "criminals" or "felons." They are bad guys. All of these terms imply that the *person* is bad or criminal, not that the person committed an *act* that was bad, criminal, or felonious. But that is not how we see our beloved brother or other family members. We see him as a full person that deserves our sympathy. Certainly, we might be annoyed, angry, or upset about his stealing. After all, we have been harmed! But we likely will consider what caused him to steal from us. (Is he struggling with money? Is he struggling with addiction? Does he need help getting a job? Does he need our love, care, and attention?) We likely are willing to consider how that brother can make it up to us to repair our relationship. And we probably will assist him in making a plan for earning a reliable paycheck, seeking substance abuse treatment and therapy, or finding a support network.

These ideas are the foundation of restorative justice. Restorative justice is not about punishing; rather, it is about repairing harms. Critical to the process is the dignity of both the person who is harmed and the person who has done the harm. Our current prison system does little to repair the harm caused. Sometimes, the victim or victim's family feels relief that the person is imprisoned. It can be a powerful recognition that a harm occurred. But oftentimes, imprisonment solves nothing. It does not even require an apology or any type of repair to the people harmed.

Restorative justice aims to bring victim and perpetrator (and sometimes others in the community) together to share what happened, who was harmed, and how the perpetrator can repair the harms that they caused. Ultimately, the goal of a restorative justice process is for the perpetrator to take responsibility for their actions and for the person harmed to be empowered in the process.

Restorative justice contrasts to our typical system of *retributive* justice, which focuses primarily on punishment for the perpetrator of harm. The criminal legal system in the United States is based on this concept. But retributive justice can disempower victims and does not actually attend to the victim's needs or require that the perpetrator takes responsibility for their actions. A review of the evidence comparing restorative justice practices with retributive justice practices showed that restorative justice can reduce repeat offending, encourage people to report harms, reduce posttraumatic stress experienced by victims, increase satisfaction by victims and perpetrators, and overall reduce costs.[154]

In Colorado's 11th judicial district, they are experimenting with restorative justice practices to divert young people from the criminal legal system. After an incident of harm occurs, the district court can refer the case to a Full Circle Restorative Justice Diversion Program.[155] At that point, the Full Circle program would invite the victim or harmed person and the responsible person into a restorative justice process. Each person has the option to refuse, and the case will be referred back to the court. But, if both parties agree, the Full Circle program will first meet separately with the victim/harmed person and the responsible person to better understand their experience and to determine if a restorative process is a good fit. If it is, they will then bring them together in a group session facilitated by a trained restorative justice facilitator. That meeting is intended to allow the victim to share the impact of the harm and the responsible person to share what caused the incident to occur. The session is intended to produce an agreement between the two parties about how the responsible person can repair the harm and restore the relationship. The agreements are specific and time-bound. If the responsible party follows the agreements, their case will be dropped from the judicial district, and they would not have a criminal record. The Full Circle process is based on restorative justice principles of "relationship, respect, responsibility, repair, and reintegration." One of the victims who participated said, "Although I was initially hesitant, the Full Circle advocate supported me to find my voice. I found the courage to move forward and discover a resilience I didn't know I had."[155]

As shown with this example, restorative justice practices can divert people from prison or juvenile detention centers. The United States has the highest incarceration rate in the entire world, with 664 people imprisoned for every 100,000. In Louisiana and Mississippi, the rate is even higher, with over 1,000 people incarcerated per 100,000, which is equivalent to 1% of their population.[156] So what would it look like if we moved away from such a system where we used prisons as our default solution when a harm was committed?

While many prison abolitionists are working to envision and build a world without prisons at all, there are no countries (yet) that have fully adopted that model. One case worth noting, however, is the Netherlands, which incarcerates a dramatically lower proportion of its population. In 2019, the Netherlands closed 13 prisons because they were not being used.[157] The country's incarceration rate is 63 per 100,000, which is about 10% of the rate in the United States.[156] Part of this decline is due to diverting people from jails and into community service programs; another part is diverting people into mental health services to address root causes. Notably, the Netherlands has a much more robust social safety net system that helps meet people's basic needs. Meeting basic needs related to health, housing, and food is a simple strategy to keep people from committing harms in the first place.

New York and New Jersey are states that have reduced their prison populations—though not to the same extent as the Netherlands. Between 1999 and 2012, they lowered their prison populations by 26%, despite the fact that nationwide, the state prison population increased by 10% in the same period. They did this by diverting felony drug convictions to treatment programs, reducing mandatory sentencing, and making it easier for prisoners to get parole.[158]

Taking a more restorative justice approach rather than retributive justice (i.e., revenge) is not about avoiding accountability. It is an alternative path to accountability. And as an added benefit, the approach adopts more of a prevention mindset: How do we prevent such things from happening again? The evidence shows that restorative justice practices can be more successful than retributive justice at preventing recidivism and helping to heal. A meta-analysis of research on restorative justice conferences (like the Full Circle example) found that people who were randomly assigned to these conferences instead of receiving a regular punishment were less likely to commit another offense. Across studies in the meta-analysis, people who went through a restorative justice conference had between 7% and 45% fewer repeat convictions or arrests.[159]

If we truly treat everyone in our society as humans, including those who cause harm, we can imagine new systems that will actually prevent harms in the first place and provide care and resources—instead of merely punishment—for those who cause harm. Next, we will look at how this might change our approach to public safety.

CHAPTER 7

Better Public Safety

What Makes Us Feel Safe?

My town of Ann Arbor, Michigan, often finds itself near the top of internet lists on the "best place to live for families." Fortune Magazine ranked it number 2 in 2022.[160] Livability.com named it number 2 in 2022.[161] Niche.com named it number 7 in 2023.[162] Many who live here consider the city to be safe, friendly, and welcoming. But, like elsewhere in America, your experience of safety depends on who you are.

In 2014, Ann Arbor police responded to a 911 call about a domestic disturbance at a home about a mile from where I currently live. Approximately 10 seconds after arriving on the scene, the Ann Arbor police officer fatally shot Aura Rosser, a 40-year-old artist and mother of three children. The police officer was white, and Aura Rosser was Black. While the police alleged that Rosser approached them with a knife in hand, the immediate response was firing a bullet into her chest rather than the use of de-escalation tactics.[163] Was it safe, friendly, and welcoming for someone like Rosser if ultimately the people who are ostensibly there to "serve and protect" took her life?

Protests erupted in Ann Arbor after Rosser's death, and community members demanded accountability. But the scene played out in Ann Arbor largely as it has played out in countless other cities across the United States: the prosecutor declined to bring any charges against David Ried, the police officer who shot Rosser, and he still patrols Ann Arbor. The prosecutor argued that Ried acted exactly as he should have.[164]

This event in Ann Arbor occurred just a few months after the shooting of Michael Brown in August 2014 by police officer Darren Wilson in Ferguson, Missouri. That death sparked outrage and a protest movement that has questioned the role of police in keeping a community safe. If police had been able to stop killing people, and Black men in particular, after that moment the movement may have lost steam. But, tragically, police across the United States continued to kill people, mostly with impunity. In fact, police killings are trending upward, with more people killed by police in 2024 (1,252), 2023 (1,247), 2022 (1,201), and 2021 (1,147) than in any other year in the previous decade.[165] Since the Ferguson uprising, police have killed over 1,000 people per year.[165]

The movement to question the role of police in our communities hit a crescendo in 2020, after news of the murders of George Floyd and Breonna Taylor at the hands of police spread across the world. In the case of George Floyd, he was murdered by Minneapolis police over a $20 counterfeit bill.[166] In the case of Breonna Taylor, she was murdered when Louisville police officers dressed in plain clothes broke into her house in the middle of the night.[167] Is this the best version of public safety we can imagine?

*   *   *

While people commonly targeted by police have been sounding the alarm for decades, there has been wider recognition that our system of policing may not be the most effective way to ensure that all members of society are safe and able to thrive. At its worst, some members of society are dying because of police action. Many others are injured, harassed, or get ensnared into our criminal legal system in ruinous ways because of our policing systems. In addition to these direct harms, more broadly, the system contributes to inequalities in society and fuels distrust.

Some people are quick to argue that a few officers who are "bad apples" should not make us question the whole system. But the question of whether or not individual police officers are good or bad people distracts from the more important question of whether this *system* is the best designed solution to keep people safe. Are our local governments asking police departments and officers to do something that causes harm to our communities? Over the last century, our communities have largely created institutions of policing that have become increasingly militarized and have prioritized protecting wealth and people with some degree of power. As a society, we have enabled a culture of impunity for law enforcement—and public policies that support a lack of accountability for police—and funded the militarization with a focus on protecting privileged members of our community, regardless of the consequences for marginalized groups.

What happened in Ann Arbor, Ferguson, Louisville, Minneapolis, and thousands of other places invites us to question the public safety policies and systems that we have in place. All too often, officers are taking lives when they are responding in ways that they were trained. In nearly all cases of police killings, our legal system looks at what the officer's actions were and responds that they were acting exactly how they were supposed to. But is this harm to individuals and communities actually necessary for public safety? Or, could we imagine alternative policies and systems?

* * *

Let us first take a look at the documented harms that our current system causes. Our public safety policies are a key pathway to incarceration, which does its own harm to individuals and communities. But our system of policing has its own unique impact on who lives, who dies, and who thrives. Public safety policies are typically seen as responding to social issues related to crime, but in the United States, the emphasis is on using law enforcement to resolve these issues. Law enforcement agencies include local and state police. There are also federal law enforcement agencies such as Immigration and Customs Enforcement (ICE), the US Border Patrol, the Drug Enforcement Administration, and others. Our public policies in this area shape how much funding these agencies receive, which weapons they can use against residents and when, and what level of impunity they have for harms they cause.

Public safety policies in the United States heavily fund law enforcement officers who carry weapons that they are legally authorized to use, creating an environment where over 1,000 people are killed and over 50,000 young people are injured each year by law enforcement.[168] Black, Latino, and Native American people—as well as those who are homeless, mentally ill, or transgender/nonbinary—are much more likely to experience these deaths or injuries. In fact, Black men have a 1 in 1,000 chance of being killed by police in their lifetime (it is the 6th leading cause of death for young Black men). By comparison, other men have a 1 in 2,000 chance.[169] Women, trans, and nonbinary individuals are also killed and injured each year, in addition to being the regular targets of sexual violence by police, though precise statistics can be harder to ascertain.[170] These numbers show that the system created to promote safety is causing a lot of collateral damage to people within our communities.

Aside from physical or sexual violence perpetrated by police, other actions such as police surveillance, street stops, or verbal harassment can affect the health and well-being of our communities in several ways. These tactics are linked to heightened depressive symptoms and higher rates of trauma, anxiety, and posttraumatic stress, particularly among young men.[171] Youth of color and urban teens who are exposed to either aggressive policing practices or vicarious police contact exhibit both lower educational performance and achievement.[172,173] Negative encounters with law enforcement are also linked to heightened mistrust and avoidance of health care institutions.[174,175] People exposed to hostile policing practices have shorter telomere lengths—a biological marker of cellular aging associated with premature death and disability—and research has shown this effect is most pronounced for Black men.[176] These policing tactics not only directly harm the people they are used against, but they have spillover effects on their neighbors.[177] Recent evidence shows that residing in a neighborhood where police have recently killed someone makes individuals more likely to have high blood pressure and other disease risk factors.[178]

Beyond local law enforcement, actions taken by the Border Patrol or by ICE can cause significant harms. Some of my own research with immigrant communities has shown that deportation and detention tactics can lead immigrant families to protect themselves by not leaving their house, causing them to neglect preventive health care and avoid trips to the grocery or pharmacy or engagement with their community.[179] Scholar William Lopez wrote the book *Separated* to humanize the situation and help us understand how the actions of law enforcement can hurt immigrant families and the communities they live in.[180] The harms of our current approach touch many people and aspects of community life.

*   *   *

As I was writing this chapter at a local coffeeshop in Ann Arbor, I sat next to two college students who were casually talking about underage drinking and the drug use going on in their dorm at the university where I teach. Notably absent from their conversation was any mention of police raids or police surveillance of their dorm to curtail these violations of the law. Contrast this with police raids and surveillance of public housing complexes.

The absence of police raids at college dorms is largely because our public policies have given law enforcement officers extraordinary discretion over which violations of law they target. This discretion is similar to those enjoyed by judges and prosecutors in the criminal justice system. Police can choose who they arrest and who they let go along their way.[181] They can choose whether they surveil a public housing complex or a college dorm. They can choose whether to direct their vast resources toward enforcing laws against a corporation stealing wages from workers or toward people stealing diapers and medicine.

In 2022, the New York Police Department proudly reported on social media that it had conducted a sting operation that arrested 23 individuals and recovered stolen goods. Then came an outcry when the public learned (from a photo the NYPD posted) that the average amount each person stole was less than $100, and the stolen items were primarily diapers and medicine.[182] This began a public discussion about whether taxpayer support of this type of sting operation made sense or if taxpayer money could have been directed to helping poor people afford things like diapers and medicine. If we are trying to create safety for people, is this the best and most cost-effective approach?

* * *

Law enforcement agencies are incredibly well funded and eat up a significant amount of city budgets. Despite the attention given to calls to "defund the police," studies show an actual increase in the proportion of public expenditure allocated to law enforcement.[183] A 2020 study done by the Vera Institute of Justice of the 72 largest US cities showed that the median city spent 29% of its municipal budget on police, with some cities like Phoenix and Milwaukee spending over 40% of their municipal budget on local police.[184] Importantly, these dollars often come at the expense of funding cuts to education or social services. Over the past decades, cities have chosen to increase the amount of funding for police while largely leaving funding for poverty stagnant.

In 1965, President Lyndon B. Johnson and US politicians were concerned about growing crime in US cities. Johnson created the Commission on Law Enforcement and Administration of Justice to help make cities safer so that residents could live without fear of theft, violence, or other harms. The commission included lawyers, judges, prosecutors, police officials, and other leaders and studied the issue for almost 20 months. This was part of Johnson's War on Crime initiative. The commission issued a report that said: *"Warring on poverty, inadequate housing, and unemployment is warring on crime. A civil rights law is a law against crime. Money for schools is money against crime."* [185] In other words, preventing thefts, violence, and other harms is more about providing for people's basic needs rather than the actions of police or prosecutors. And yet, the United States has repeatedly chosen public policies and budgets that emphasize armed law enforcement instead of other types of resources (e.g., social workers, mental health services, education, conflict de-escalation, housing support) that promote public safety.

Historian Elizabeth Hinton has studied this phenomenon and documented it in her book *From the War on Poverty to the War on Crime.*[186] She writes that in the decades since the 1960s, the federal government has increased support to cities for policing and reduced funding for anti-poverty programs or social services. Over time, police filled the gap left by the lack of social services, sometimes quite literally. Hinton demonstrates this by sharing the true story of the community center in Washington, D.C., that was turned into a police station outpost.

Do these public policy choices in the realm of law enforcement actually lead to public safety? There is some evidence to suggest that funding for police can reduce social problems like murder, burglary, or assault. But a city would need to spend an estimated $1.3 million to $2.2 million on 10 additional police officers to prevent one murder.[187] Saving a life may certainly be worth that investment of money, but it needs to be considered alongside the collateral damage the increased police force might cause. With the goal of public safety and a thriving society, is it where the money can best be utilized? Other policy options have been shown to prevent murders and other violence at a lower cost (e.g., blighted housing and alcohol policies), and they do not come with the additional harms of law enforcement agencies.[188–190] To apply a prevention mindset to this area—to prevent problems before they start—we will need to invest in people and communities rather than systems that can cause harm.

Imagining a Better World: Policies Based on a Prevention Mindset

In 2022, I attended a Zoom workshop facilitated by Yodit Mesfin Johnson, a change-maker who pushes for equity and justice in her local communities. Yodit works in my county with nonprofit groups to help them realize their goals and better work toward equity. She was facilitating a session with a group of advocates who were working toward a different vision of public safety in our town of Ann Arbor. This work had through lines to the activism that responded to the killing of Aura Rosser by local police. Drawing on the tradition of Black radical imagination, in which "the map to a new world is in the imagination,"[16] Yodit asked us to imagine what this vision of public safety would look like, taste like, feel like, smell like. We were invited to truly swim in our imaginations and conceive of an alternative society that thought differently about how to keep people safe and whole.

When we individually thought about the things that make us feel safe, our responses were loved ones, presence of community, having food and shelter, and a sense of belonging. The presence of police did not necessarily indicate safety, and sometimes it was menacing—threatening actions that could hurt us, punish us, or intimidate us. That was even true for me, a white educated man who had only a few negative encounters with police. Their presence usually indicated that something was wrong or could go wrong. In contrast, our imagined future amplified the things that made us feel safe: tight connections with neighbors, supportive care in times of need, and the smells of cooking wafting from people's homes.

What Yodit asked us to do is something that will be vital to thinking about applying a prevention mindset to our public safety. There are versions of "safety" in this world that rely on barbed wire fences, armed guards, alarm systems, and heavy surveillance. But that safety is tenuous and has real costs for people that live within that version of safety. Instead, we need to imagine a society where the foundations of safety are based on things like love, care, connection, and provision of basic needs rather than violence, punishment, and intimidation. Go ahead. Take a minute to imagine what that would look like for you. What does your vision of community safety look like? What would you see? What would you hear? What would you smell? How would you feel?

No doubt some of you will read this and think that it is far-fetched, idealistic, and unrealistic to think that this imagined world could really exist. It is certainly a transformation from our current system, but our societies have undergone transformations before. Our current vision of safety—one dominated by policing—is less than 200 years old.[191] We may be overdue for a new approach. For most of human history, our safety did not depend on police. It depended on our neighbors, family, and connections to other humans.

* * *

Luna Hughson, an advocate for alternatives to policing, has done some of this reimagining. In 2018, as part of advocacy for a more expansive vision of safety in her local city, she created a series of "Imagine Alternatives to Policing" flyers that encouraged people shift how they think about public safety. It is a vision based more on connecting people with resources in a time of need rather than responding with punishment. Here is the text from a few of her flyers:

You don't realize [it], but your brake lights aren't working. Imagine . . . a city employee signals for you to pull over & says "hey, how about I replace those lights for you right here so no one gets hurt?" An hour later, both lights work & you're at home. Isn't that public safety?

Your friends are intoxicated & fighting but you don't want them to get in trouble. Imagine . . . you call +311 and a crisis intervention team comes to your door. 1 hour later, your friends are sleeping it off at home. Isn't that public safety?

Someone is behaving erratically & in harm's way. Imagine . . . texting a number & an unarmed urgent responder trained in behavioral and mental health comes within 5 minutes. An hour later that person is safe & getting the support they need. Isn't that public safety?

Incidents of gun violence are rising in the neighborhood. Imagine . . . a trauma informed crisis intervention team works with community activists to disarm and deescalate conflicts. People doing harm are connected to services that address the underlying problem. Isn't that public safety?[192]

Like Yodit, Luna asks us to imagine a different way to think about these incidents and a different way to respond. All of the situations described are situations where we currently ask police to respond. Police are not trained to get to the root cause of issues. The tools they have at their disposal are used to punish people rather than provide supportive care. The responses that Luna describes deliver care and support. They do not have the potential to lead to police violence and are not a pathway to prison. They are a care-first approach that values the humanity of every person involved.

As Dallas police chief David Brown said in 2016: "We're asking cops to do too much in this country. We are. Every societal failure, we put it off on the cops to solve. Not enough mental health funding, let the cops handle it. Here in Dallas we got a loose dog problem . . . let's have the cops chase loose dogs. Schools fail, let's give it to the cops. That's too much to ask."[193] Imagine what types of resources and support we could provide in our communities with a portion of the billions of dollars allocated to law enforcement agencies.

* * *

So, let's talk more concretely. How could we change policies to be more aligned with the alternative vision that Luna describes? Alternative response programs are one prime example. What are they? Simply put, they are programs that exist within cities that respond to emergencies with trained professionals or community members who are not the police. At a basic level, these programs are an "alternative" to the police. These responders do not carry guns and do not have the authority to arrest or imprison. Instead, they respond with care and supportive resources. The reality is that in most cities, police are residents' only option to get help in the emergency situations that Luna describes.

Unarmed safety programs already exist in several cities throughout the United States. I worked with my colleagues

Maren Spolum, William Lopez, and Daphne Watkins to review some of these programs and also identify key characteristics that were in line with the prevention mindset.[194] In our work, we learned that not all programs are created equal, and there is wide variation in programs that deem themselves "alternative responses."

Some programs are merely extensions of police departments where police officers receive some special training to better respond to mental health incidents. Most commonly, they implement "crisis intervention teams."[195] Almost a quarter of police departments in the United States have been trained in this model, including departments with prominent examples of police violence.

Other programs respond to incidents with police officers at their side. This type of program does not really remove the harms of policing from the equation. The fact that police are there means that the incident still could result in a shooting, tasering, harassment, intimidation, jail time, arrest records or other harms. In addition, the fact that police are co-responding means that people who do not trust the police will not use the service because they do not want to expose themselves to the potential harms associated with an encounter with armed police.

My friend and fellow organizer Ryan Henyard has been working toward a better version of public safety, and he poignantly describes this hesitancy to call the police in an episode of the podcast *Ann Arbor AF*.[196] Ryan is a Black man from Detroit who now lives in a predominantly white town in Southeast Michigan. He said, "People are afraid to call for help for a lot of different things because of the fact that it comes with an armed response. I don't wish violence upon myself, but if I were accosted in a violent incident, I wouldn't call 911. . . ." He goes on to say, "I've lived that experience where I've been robbed and have decided that it is better for my safety to not call the emergency response line. It is more likely that I will be harmed from that interaction than made whole." The presence of police is perceived as too risky for some folks in our society to utilize as a resource, and thus alternatives are needed.

Unfortunately, our review of programs across the United States showed that alternative response programs that are completely separate from the police are fairly rare (though the idea continues to expand with new programs popping up across the country). The most prominent example of such a program is the Crisis Assistance Helping Out On The Streets (CAHOOTS) program in Eugene, Oregon. Launched in 1989, it is the country's longest-running alternative response program. CAHOOTS, which operates out of the White Bird Clinic, provides mental health first response for crises involving mental illness, homelessness, and addiction. They respond to incidents with two-person teams of a medic (a nurse, paramedic, or EMT) and a crisis worker with training and experience in the mental health field. It receives 2% of the police department's budget while handling 10% of the calls that police would traditionally handle. They estimate that this program saves the city about $8.5 million annually.[197,198] CAHOOTS does still sometimes call police for backup, but this happens in less than 1% of response situations.[199]

Another example that has been somewhat modeled after CAHOOTS is the Support Team Assisted Response (STAR) program in Denver, Colorado. During the six-month pilot, research shows that there was a 34% reduction in the incidents the STAR team was designated to respond to and a reduction in the number of crimes within the geographic boundaries of the intervention. STAR was implemented in 2020 at a quarter of the cost of a police response.[200]

After assessing these different types of programs, our team published an article in the *American Journal of Public Health* that details the three characteristics that are key for an alternative response program that is equity-focused and adopts a prevention lens:

1. *It must involve directly impacted communities in the program design, implementation, oversight, and evaluation.* Best practice for any community program is that impacted communities are at the center of the design and implementation. This is crucial for building community trust and also ensuring that the program does not replicate some of the flaws of our policing system, where responders are often perceived as community outsiders. An alternative response program should follow this simple tenet: "nothing about us without us."

2. *It needs to operate independently from law enforcement agencies and the broader criminal legal system.* The most marginalized communities should feel comfortable and secure when using the alternative response program's services. This means providing an alternative means of accessing the program through a separate number, rather than relying on 911, which is often controlled by law enforcement agencies. It also means that the program exists outside the police department and has complete autonomy from the police. It should not respond with the police as a standard practice.

3. *It must secure adequate program and social service funding by diverting funds from police.* To effectively work toward a different vision of public safety, an alternative response program must be able to reduce the involvement of police while increasing the care-based safety resources it makes available to residents. This necessarily means that police budgets will have to

shrink or stagnate while more funding is diverted into alternative response programs or other evidence-based solutions for public safety.

* * *

An alternative response program is not the only way to work toward reducing the harms of policing, but it can help shift public policies and community resources toward the prevention mindset. It will also need to be accompanied by a shift in how we think about public safety as a responsibility to each other (rather than something that an agency like the police alone can guarantee). We are often taught to think in terms of bad guys and good guys. Heroes and villains. The worst mistake someone makes comes to define them.

To get to a better future, we need to stop labeling each other as our mistakes and start to think of each other as humans. That person you want to label as a felon is actually someone's son or daughter, father or mother, neighbor, or soccer coach. All people have good in them, and all people make poor choices sometimes. When we think about public safety, if we could envision the humanity and good in people—and especially consider what types of basic needs people have and how to provide it—instead of envisioning only their worst characteristics, we would come to very different policies for public safety. These fundamental shifts will take time to take root, but they have the potential to create communities where people feel safe and are better able to thrive.

* * *

Part II of this book has detailed several policy areas—health care, environment, education, criminal legal, and public safety—where a prevention mindset would help us recognize the shortsightedness of our existing policies and imagine a different set of policies that might serve us all better. These categories are not the only ones where public policy is shortsighted and even harmful.

We can think of agricultural policies where the Farm Bill largely prioritizes the profits of corporate farming rather than the health and well-being of residents.[201] It subsidizes foods that are high in sugar and low-cost fats and agricultural practices that pollute our air and water. Think about an immigration policy that targets immigrants who are filling labor needs and punishes them by detaining them without legal support, ultimately separating them from their children, family, and community.[202] Think about our economic policies; in many settings, they disadvantage labor unions or other workers and give advantages to the bankers or wealthy executives. These policies exacerbate economic inequality and create conditions where it is extremely challenging for millions of workers to prioritize health and well-being.[203] We can think about the shortsightedness of our tax policies that starve health-promoting social services and benefits by lowering taxes on wealthy individuals and protecting certain types of wealth creation from taxes.[204] And we can examine our transportation policy, where as a nation we have largely invested in an infrastructure that prioritizes individual cars rather than one that promotes walking, biking, or public transportation. These policy priorities not only make it difficult for many people without cars to access health-related resources, but they are also associated with more motor vehicle accidents and fatalities, poor mental and physical health as a result of people getting less physical activity, and an upsurge in pollution and climate change.[205]

While I have presented the policy areas as separate, they often work synergistically to create devastating results for our society, and especially poor and racially marginalized communities. Before we move into part III, which focuses on the *action* we can take, we need to spend a bit more time reflecting, specifically on the histories that created the world as we know it in present day.

CHAPTER 8

Looking Back to Look Forward

Studying history aims to loosen the grip of the past. It enables us to turn our head this way and that, and begin to notice possibilities.

—Yuval Noah Harari, *Homo Deus: A Brief History of Tomorrow*

You know that saying, "History is written by victors"? Who do you think of when you hear that phrase? The Roman empire? European kings? It is also important to think about the more recent past and the United States and its "victors." Most often in US history, those victors have been white land-owning men with political or financial power. It is only through the eyes of these white victors that we can talk about the early decades of US history without referring to the genocide of Indigenous peoples in North America. It is only through the eyes of white victors that we can frame the Civil Rights Movement as ending in the 1960s with all the needed reforms. And it is only through the eyes of white victors that we can view the mistakes of the past through a lens of ignorance rather than an effort to build wealth by a wealthy white decision-makers.

In recent years, there are active efforts by policymakers to prohibit teaching history that is written from the perspective of marginalized communities or tarnishes the image of the United

States.[206,207] Indeed, it is the "victors" of recent elections who are trying to make decisions about what our history is. But how can our perspective shift when we put the history of marginalized groups at the center? It can help us better get at the root cause of vast inequities in our society.

Studying these painful histories is not simply to criticize and tarnish the United States. It is in service of identifying the transformation that is needed to work toward a different society. There are so many strengths of the United States, its people, and its government that can be built on to make a better society where all people can thrive. But a lot of the good is connected with the bad. Our wealth and opportunities for many would not have been possible without stealing land from Indigenous Americans and creating an exploited class of people through chattel slavery, Jim Crow laws, and exclusionary immigration policies. As a country, the United States is a work in progress with much potential and much to atone for and redress. We are at a critical moment in our country where our full history is being obscured, and there are efforts to return us to some of the harmful choices of our past.

So, how *did* we get here? How did we get to this point in time with these public policies and these unjust and inequitable outcomes across society? We need to go back centuries to understand the foundations of how our society is structured, who got to make decisions, and what those decisions were. Before we can strategize how to take action, we need to understand the historical roots.

This chapter is not a comprehensive history, but it will help us to think about the choices and paths our society has taken over the years. It focuses on some of the root causes of the racial inequities that are pervasive in the United States. As we saw in prior chapters, our policy choices have created stark racial inequities across a range of outcomes. Once we look back into history and see all the choices we made to get to our present day, it becomes easier to understand our current moment. And it becomes easier to envision and imagine alternative paths toward a more equitable and better future.

Ahistorical perspectives are incomplete. As we can see from the Flint water crisis example, the story is insufficient if we don't look at what happened in the past to shape the crisis. If we don't account for history, not only do we misunderstand the present, we also close doors in our imagination. Journalist and author Nikole Hannah-Jones wrote a powerful essay arguing for reparations for Black Americans: *"When it comes to truly explaining racial injustice in this country, the table should never be set quickly: There is too much to know, and yet we aggressively choose not to know it."*[208] Our society "aggressively chooses not to know it" because it is disruptive to the present-day status quo. But understanding our history is about looking at root causes. It is an essential component of a prevention mindset.

* * *

To understand policies in the United States, we have to first examine the concept of race in our society. When you think about race, do you think of it as something that is natural/biological or man-made? A lot of folks struggle with this question because they think they are seeing "biology" when they see someone's skin color, hair type, or their facial features. But the reality is that the biology behind those features are not necessarily what define race. Race is a set of groupings that societies have placed onto people that were created by people (i.e., socially constructed). The specific color or phenotype of your skin may be based on your biological makeup, but what that color means and how it shapes your experience of the world is something humans created.

The Human Genome Project mapped the genes of *Homo sapiens* and found that there were no genetic markers for what US society and the broader world thinks of as "races."[209] You cannot look at someone's genes and know with certainty what race they are. That is because genes do not decide racial categories—people do.

Another way that we know that race is not biological but something that humans invented is that ideas of race, and who is considered "white," have shifted over time and vary by context. In other words, who is considered white in the United States in the 21st century is very different from who was considered white 200 years ago. For example, Irish immigrants were initially considered to be a different race than English immigrants.[210] Like almost all "racial science," it was done with the intent to emphasize English superiority over this other group. Similarly, someone considered Black in one country may be considered a different race in a different country.[211] For example, the United States and South Africa are two different cultural contexts, and who gets categorized as Black in each context is different.[212] It has been determined not by biology but by what powerful people in each context say it is. Even though it is not biological, race still has very real impacts because of its role in creating social hierarchies in these societies.

* * *

OK, so if it is invented, who invented it? We need to go back about 600 years. Historian Dr. Ibram X. Kendi writes in detail about this moment in his National Book Award–winning *Stamped from the Beginning: The Definitive History of Racist Ideas in America*.[213] Fifteenth-century European kings were trying to build wealth by extracting resources from other regions. During this period, slavery was common, but not yet based on "race" or ancestry. People from Europe, Africa, and Asia were enslaved. Enslavers thought of enslaved people as inferior to their own group, but it was not necessarily based on racial categories.

In 1453, the king of Portugal wanted to glorify and justify the Portuguese colonizers who were enslaving Africans. So, he commissioned a book by Gomez de Zurara. This author lumped light- and dark-skinned Africans into one singular category. Previously, people were considered by their ethnicity or religion. He described this new large and varied category of people as "beasts." He further justified the enslavement of African people by saying that it was needed to bring them closer to Christianity, the main religion practiced in Portugal.

De Zurara is credited with first creating the idea of race, though many more would add to it over time. Many Europeans eagerly adopted this viewpoint and built on it to justify their own feeling of superiority and the benefits they received as a result.[213,214] Today, we see widespread disparities across the world based on the racial categories that were invented centuries ago.

The racist ideas that were being created in Europe eventually found their way to the Americas and what we now call the United States. Colonizers from Europe were coming to the North American shores with racist ideas that Africans and Europeans were fundamentally different. As they began to create governments and institutions in the US colonies, they started to put these racist ideas into their public policies.

Indentured servants—those that were servants for someone until they paid off their debt—were a key labor source in the new US colonies.[215] In 1640 Virginia, an indentured servant originally from Africa, John Punch, attempted to escape servitude alongside two indentured servants originally from Europe. After being caught, the Europeans servants had four years added to their servitude while John Punch was punished with lifetime servitude.[216] This was the first time the idea of perpetual servitude for Africans was written into law and a legal distinction was made based on race in the US colonies.*

---

* The text from the ruling on John Punch reads: "One called Victor, a Dutchman, the other a Scotchman called James Gregory, shall first serve out their times with their master according to their Indentures, and one

In 1682, Virginia's legislature, the House of Burgesses, explicitly limited citizenship to the new territory to only Europeans. Further, they wrote into law that "Negroes, Moors, Mollatoes, and Indians" are "slaves to all intents and purposes."[217] In 1691, they used "white" as a descriptor for Europeans for the first time in a law defining citizenship.[218] Before this, the concept of white and Black (or "Negroes") was not written into law. But this was only the beginning. Race would become a key feature of our law for the following centuries.

This history, starting in Europe, brought racial categories into the US context and created vast inequities between Black and white residents who were coming—or being forced to come—to the United States. But what about the people who were already here?

* * *

The Native Americans had to contend with settler colonialism in the land they lived on and stewarded. Settler colonialism is an ongoing system of power that perpetuates the genocide and repression of Indigenous peoples, and it normalizes the continuous settler occupation and exploits Indigenous lands and resources.[219] The very first Europeans to come to North America were there to discover trade routes and claim land to grow their wealth.

The common history of "explorers" is riddled with stories of European men who "brought their ship upon [insert large swath of North American land already inhabited] and claimed that land for King [insert extremely wealthy monarch in

---

whole year apiece after the time of their service is expired by their said indentures in recompense of his loss sustained by their absence, and after that service to their said master is expired, to serve the colony for three whole years apiece. And that the third being a negro named John Punch shall serve his said master or his assigns for the time of his natural life here or elsewhere."

Europe]." My favorite of these stories is Vasco Núñez de Balboa, who was the first European colonizer to see what we now call the Pacific Ocean. He saw it and claimed the ocean and *all of its shores*—all 352 quintillion gallons in that ocean and land of four continents—for Spain.[220] Of course, that notion is absurd, but such was the hubris, ignorance, and greed of the Europeans stepping onto lands of Indigenous peoples in North America.

Eventually, the English began setting up more and more colonies and settlements in the present-day United States. Those settlements required pushing Indigenous peoples off their land. After the creation of the United States of America, the government and its European residents began to see it as their "manifest destiny" to seize land across the North American continent.[221]

European settlers and the US government took land through numerous strategies.[222] Sometimes they used outright violence and war, slaughtering Native American families before taking their land.[223] In other cases, they squatted on land that had been used by Native families.[224] Sometimes, they used coercive strategies to pay, trade, or negotiate with Native communities for their land.[225] And sometimes they used biased legal rulings to remove tribal land rights.[226]

Perhaps the most famous example of this removal is the Indian Removal Act and the resulting Trail of Tears. Under the Andrew Jackson administration, Congress passed the Indian Removal Act in 1830 with the goal of forcing Native Americans living on their ancestral lands in the southeastern United States to move into US territories west of the Mississippi.[227] When the law was passed, there were about 125,000 Native Americans living on millions of acres of land in the Southeast.[228] European settlers wanted to use this land to have enslaved Africans plant and harvest cotton and grow their fortune. To enable this wealth creation through exploitation of enslaved African people, the US government forced thousands of Native Americans off their land. The Trail of Tears refers to the forced march from their homeland to territory in present-day Oklahoma. Many historians estimate that thousands of Native Americans died during the journey or as part of being forced off their land.[229]

The Native communities tried to start a new life in the "Indian Territory" that was supposed to be theirs. But just a half century later, white settlers continued to move further and further west, and ultimately Oklahoma was the site of more settler encroachment. In 1907, Oklahoma was established as a state controlled by white settlers.

There is an interactive map called "Invasion of America."[230] It catalogs all the different treaties and executive orders that established reservations for Native Americans or took them away. You can follow how the US government took *1.5 billion* acres of land from Native communities between 1776 and 1890.

Aside from taking land, the US government tried to force Native Americans to adopt their culture and customs. Most egregiously, they would force children from Native families to attend boarding schools. The Bureau of Indian Affairs had a "Civilization Division" that promoted forced assimilation through boarding schools.[231] The government operated over 100 boarding schools specifically for Native American children both on and off reservation land.[232] There was rampant abuse within the schools, and the children were forced to adopt white European culture.

This brings us to the idea of genocide. Patrick Wolfe is a prominent anthropologist who writes that "the question of genocide is never far from discussions of settler colonialism. Land is life— or at least, land is necessary for life."[233]

The UN Genocide Convention declares several acts as genocide if "committed with intent to destroy, in whole or in part, a national, ethnical, racial or religious group."[234] This definition includes:

- Killing members of the group or causing serious bodily or mental harm
- Deliberately inflicting conditions of life calculated to bring about destruction in whole or part.
- Forcibly transferring children of the group to another group

The US government participated in killing and causing serious harm to Indigenous people, depriving them of life-giving resources, and forcibly transferring their children into harmful European boarding schools. Contemporary research shows that this unacknowledged genocide in our history has resulted in poor mental health and chronic disease within Native American communities, attributed to their being disconnected from their culture and land.[235,236] Native Americans pushed back against this encroachment and genocide every step of the way and continue to fight for their culture and way of life in the present day. This history underscores the ways that our policies from the beginning have prioritized the well-being of some at the expense of others.

* * *

The United States created classifications for white and Black that created a power hierarchy, and settlers subjugated and sought to eliminate Native Americans from their ancestral homeland. But what about the newcomers who were coming from places like Asia or Latin America?

For the first part of US history, the categories of people were primarily white, Black, and "Indian." The Naturalization Act of 1790 stated that US citizenship could be given to "any alien, being a free white person."[237] Citizenship—and thus rights—were reserved for white people explicitly. That changed with the 14th Amendment, ratified in 1868 in the aftermath of the Civil War, which granted citizenship to all persons "born or naturalized in the United States."[238] The constitutional amendment was intended to grant citizenship to Black residents who had been formerly enslaved. Revisions to this law in 1870 made it even more explicit by saying naturalization is limited to "aliens being free white persons, and to aliens of African nativity and to persons of African descent."[239] Citizenship and its benefits were only available to whites and Blacks. To put an exclamation point on it, the 1882 Chinese Exclusion Act banned immigration and naturalization of Chinese people.[239] At the time, there were thousands of Chinese coming to the West Coast to work on a key new feature of the US economy: building out the transcontinental railroads.

As more and more immigrants came into the United States in the latter part of the 19th century, it caused the government to create more formalized rules and processes for how someone could become a citizen. The Naturalization Act of 1906 required immigrants to appeal to a federal court for citizenship. Because you had to be either Black or white to be a naturalized citizen, immigrants found themselves trying to prove to courts that they were white to gain citizenship. Why didn't they try to prove to the courts that they were Black? Given the racism throughout society, being deemed Black in America was not considered the same prize and access to upward mobility that being white in America was.[240] So when immigrants were trying to gain naturalization, they were arguing that they were white.

Two key court cases helped to further establish whiteness within the law. The first important case was *Ozawa v. United States* (1922), in which Takao Ozawa from Japan argued he should be classified as white because he had light skin, spoke English at home, and attended American schools and churches.[239,241] In 1922, the Supreme Court was a group of white men with European heritage, just as it had been every single year before and for 45 or more years in the future. This group of white men ruled that Ozawa was not white because white means "Caucasian," and Ozawa was Asian. The second case, *Thind v. United States* (1923) took place the year after the Ozawa case.[239,241] The court had just ruled that to be deemed white you had to be "Caucasian." Baghat Thind, from India, was originally from the Caucasus Mountains, so he argued to the Supreme Court that he was white based on their ruling in the Ozawa case. But, predictably, the men on the Supreme Court wriggled out of that argument by declaring that the "common man" would not view Thind as white.

It was through these efforts that the court played a role in defining whiteness and therefore who had access to the resources and benefits of citizenship in the United States. When we say that race is a socially constructed concept, it is these court cases—and this specific group of white men—that put into place some of the scaffolding that defines racial categories in society to this day.

Being legally white meant access to power and resources, so the US government limited who could be white. Over time, immigrants were racialized into categories that broke the Black/white/Native American racial system. Limiting the rights of immigrant groups allowed whites to retain power and build wealth with low-cost immigrant labor. Throughout US history, and even into our present day, immigrants have been recruited into the United States as a source of cheap labor (immigrants are also sometimes recruited for high-skilled and high-pay work). The Bracero program recruited 4.5 million laborers from Latin America to work in the United States but provided limited pay, resources, and worker protections.[242,243] Today, undocumented laborers fill a much-needed demand for cheap labor but earn low

wages, have no protections of citizenship, and are actively targeted by law enforcement.[244] Despite creating wealth for the
United States, immigrants have often been denied rights, safe
working and living conditions, and have been relegated to
second-class status.

* * *

We can also turn our attention toward a slightly more recent history of inequitable public policies. When people hear the term
"affirmative action," most people think of efforts to hire people of
color or women over the past decades. It was coined in 1961 to
promote fair hiring and employment for people that had been
historically discriminated against because of their race, ethnicity, or religion.[245] However, major wealth-building policies in the
20th century have largely benefited white Americans, not racially marginalized communities. This caused the scholar and
historian Ira Katznelson to coin the phrase "affirmative action
for whites," to refer to the ways that the United States government funded public policies that affirmatively advantaged and
advanced the prosperity of white people.[246] So what were these
policies?

In 1944, the GI Bill was passed to provide resources for
soldiers returning from World War II. It provided things like
low-cost mortgages, low-interest business loans, tuition support,
and unemployment benefits. All of these benefits were tremendous opportunities for individuals to invest in themselves and
build wealth. The bill is widely touted as creating a robust middle
class and creating an economic boom in the postwar period.[247]
But, as a scholar of this issue, Katznelson has written that there
was "no greater instrument for widening an already huge racial
gap in postwar America than the GI Bill."[246]

The GI Bill was "race-neutral," meaning that there were no
race-based exclusions written into the law. It should have been
fully available to any person of any race or ethnicity who had

served in World War II. But many of the 1.2 million Black veterans struggled to access the benefits.[246,248] Why? These funds were often distributed at the local level or by local institutions, and racism was rampant. The federal government was lax with oversight to stop the discrimination. Many banks refused to give loans to Black veterans, and some universities refused to admit Black applicants. In practice, white veterans benefited the most from this bill.

Another program that created affirmative action for white Americans was government-insured mortgages, made available through the New Deal, that helped people buy homes. Since home ownership is a big part of wealth creation in the United States, this government support was crucial. But the government would not grant mortgages in certain neighborhoods through its program of redlining neighborhoods.

Redlining was a process by which the Home Owners' Loan Corporation (HOLC)—a government-sponsored corporation created by the New Deal—devised maps that rated neighborhoods based on their risk for mortgage foreclosure. Majority Black neighborhoods were often designated as "hazardous" or highly risky merely because Black people lived there.[249] These maps were used by the government to decide who could get government-backed loans; eventually, they were used by private banks as well.[250]

The result was that Black homebuyers could not get a mortgage. These redlined neighborhoods deemed hazardous received little investment, which further exacerbated neighborhood segregation. Given the role that these maps played in determining who ultimately got mortgages, it meant that many Black homeowners could not obtain a mortgage to purchase a home and thus build wealth by growing property values. The maps entrenched the residential segregation that existed in the 1930s and, in many cases, made it much worse.

The housing segregation perpetuated through the redlining maps (and more broadly by Jim Crow segregation and other forms of forced segregation) has created cities and communities where the resources are inequitably distributed. Resources are concentrated in the areas that are more likely to have white homeowners, and as a result, those property values are much higher. This substantially contributes to the racial wealth gap we see in today's society.[251]

Health outcomes map onto historical redlining. When we look at health by neighborhood in the present day, we see that historically redlined neighborhoods are often the ones that have the poorest health.[252] As an example, researchers from the University of Maryland showed that, after controlling for factors like neighborhood median income and racial makeup, people who were from neighborhoods that had been historically redlined had a life expectancy that was five years shorter than those living in areas that had been designated blue ("still desirable") or green ("best").[253]

Affirmative action for whites meant that for much of the 20th century, wealth creation opportunities in this country were more available to white residents. Today's racial wealth gap and health gap can be traced back to these policies. This history cannot be ignored when looking at how to address present-day issues.

*   *   *

Our more recent history also shapes the present day. In the 1960s, civil rights policies were passed, and there were hopes for greater racial equity, but a backlash was brewing. The civil rights protections and racial unrest of the 1960s also led to the war on drugs. In 1971, President Richard Nixon labeled drug abuse as "public enemy number one" in a press conference and said that "in order to fight and defeat this enemy, it is necessary to wage a new, all-out offensive."[254] That statement led to the what came to be known as the war on drugs, which is still ongoing as of 2024. To date, the United States has spent over $1 trillion combating drug abuse, including $39 billion in fiscal year 2022.[255] But this set of public policies and budget allocations have had devastating effects on some marginalized communities.

Those harms are not necessarily *unintended* consequences. Nixon's domestic policy chief John Ehrlichman was interviewed by a journalist in 1994 about drug policies, and he candidly revealed the following:

> You want to know what this was really all about? The Nixon campaign in 1968, and the Nixon White House after that, had two enemies: the antiwar left and Black people. . . . We knew we couldn't make it illegal to be either against the war or Black, but by getting the public to associate the hippies with marijuana and Blacks with heroin, and then criminalizing both heavily, we could disrupt those communities. We could arrest their leaders, raid their homes, break up their meetings, and vilify them night after night on the evening news. Did we know we were lying about the drugs? Of course we did.[256]

This statement by Ehrlichman confirmed what many had long suspected: the war on drugs has its origins in racist policies, and it architects were intentional about the harms that they were inflicting on Black communities. Indeed, a Brookings Institute report also confirms it: "Despite its dramatic policy failures, the War on Drugs has been wildly successful in one specific area: institutionalizing racism. The drug war was built on a foundation of racism and xenophobia."[257]

How did the war on drugs institutionalize racism? By criminalizing drug use and connecting it to harsh prison sentences, the drug war enabled a form of social control in society. This has been documented extensively, most notably in the book *The New*

Jim Crow by Michelle Alexander. Alexander documents how drug laws were not evenly enforced across the population; rather, enforcement officers specifically targeted Black communities and other people of color through racial profiling practices.[258] Over the decades, the legal and human rights of residents—including suspects and defendants—were curtailed while police and law enforcement gained more funding and power. The institutionalized racism is apparent in the drastically different mandatory sentences given to people who used crack cocaine (more commonly used by Black residents) compared to those who used powder cocaine (more commonly used by white residents).[259] The differential enforcement and punishment of drug laws led to conditions where Black residents and other people of color were much more likely to be surveilled, arrested, convicted, imprisoned, and have felony records than their white counterparts, despite equal levels of drug use by both populations.[258,260] The bias and racism is baked into the system at multiple levels and has a huge impact on the outcomes for people of color.

Thankfully, there is growing recognition of the harms of the war on drugs. *The New Jim Crow* emphasizes how drug war policies helped to create a new racial regime, another iteration of structural racism that followed chattel slavery and then Jim Crow.[258] While Alexander's book illuminated how the war on drugs has contributed to mass incarceration and shift the perception for many segments of the American public, it has not halted the war on drugs.

In June 2023, human rights experts at the United Nations released a statement urging countries, including the United States, to end the war on drugs:

> The international community must replace punishment with support and promote policies that respect, protect and fulfill the rights of all. . . . The "war on drugs" may be understood to a significant

extent as a war on people. Its impact has been greatest on those who live in poverty, and it frequently overlaps with discrimination directed at marginalised groups, minorities and Indigenous Peoples.[261]

In the US context, these policies have led to irreparable harm related to the surveillance, harassment, detention, incarceration, and violation of human rights of marginalized communities. While some efforts—such as reducing the disparity in sentencing between crack and powder cocaine and reducing excessive prison sentences—have stopped some harmful aspects of the war on drugs, its effects are still being strongly felt across marginalized communities and play an important role in preventing some people and communities from thriving.[262,263]

*   *   *

This chapter has covered a sliver of our history and focused on some of the root causes of inequities within our society. The materials listed in the appendix at the end of this book will give readers an even deeper understanding of the context surrounding these concepts.

Understanding this history is critical for identifying where we go next. The following chapters move into action. Reflecting on this history, as well as the policies we are currently making and the options for alternative paths, what can we concretely do to make a better world possible?

PART III

Action

CHAPTER 9

Getting to Prevention-Minded Public Policy

> All the great transformations that society undergo rely on the low-key scheming of everyday people.
> —Ruha Benjamin

Part II unpacked how our current policies do not use a prevention mindset and explained the historical origins of our current inequities. It also gave concrete examples of policies that could transform how we structure our society. But there are many people—you might be one of them—who feel hopeless that we can actually make meaningful change in our society.

The word *sclerotic*—which means "becoming rigid and unresponsive; losing the ability to adapt"—is frequently tossed around to describe the US Congress, the institution primarily responsible for changing our laws.[264] Further, rampant executive orders and gutting of federal programs and protections recently are backtracking on issues of equity and justice.[265] So many of our existing laws—and those being newly enacted—are *not* using a prevention mindset. They do not identify the root cause, prioritize primary prevention, or focus on the needs of affected groups. It is easy to feel like we are headed down the wrong path and that there is no hope for transformative change.

But, as activist Mariame Kaba says, "Hope is a discipline." What this quote means to me is that we need to work hard to keep our hope that a better world is possible. Hope is not about being unrealistic and living in a fantasy world. Rather, it about drawing strength and hope from the powerful examples of transformation that have occurred throughout our history when communities come together, organize, and push for change.

I also draw hope from thinking about time frames. If we are acting now for seven generations in the future, it is easier for me to be hopeful. Can we take steps toward solving our colossal and sticky problems so that our great-great-great-great-great grandchildren can live in a world free from gun violence, prisons, and structural racism, where all people are cared for and have the opportunity to thrive? We do not have to solve it all in my lifetime, but we have to lay the foundation.

The Detroit-based nonprofit Civilla has a way of setting strategic intentions that it refers to as 10-3-1-3. As Civilla's website describes it: "10 years, 3 years, 1 year, 3 months. We set goals across each of these timelines, enabling individuals to put their unique strengths to work towards a common vision. The 10-3-1-3 framework creates a shared purpose for our team and ensures our long-term visions are connected to short-term actions."[266] Connecting long-term vision to short-term actions is exactly what we need to do. For Civilla, at the scale of an organization, 10-year planning may be the longest range that is feasible and realistic. But, when we are aiming to transform our world, I might suggest we consider pushing the model out a bit: 100-30-10-3-1. Where do we want to be as a society in 100 years? What does that mean we need to accomplish by the next generation (30 years)? If that is the case, what is the groundwork that we need to lay in the next 10 years? Three years? And finally, what do we need to do *right now*, within the next year, to set all of this in motion?

If we feel like we need to solve the issues of our time in the next year or two, it is easy to get extremely overwhelmed. Don't get me wrong. We should feel a sense of urgency about protecting people in harm's way, the climate crisis, new iterations of institutionalized racism, and other threats to our health and well-being. But how can we think creatively about taking the smaller steps to where we need to go? How can we take action now to set the stage for bigger transformation?

* * *

The story of Katey Fahey is an example of taking action to tackle the root causes of problems, and it is an example that gives me hope. In 2016 (and again in 2024), my home state of Michigan was part of the crumbling "blue wall" that awarded our electoral college votes to Donald Trump. Barack Obama had won Michigan's electoral votes by a 10 percentage point margin in 2012, and the Democratic presidential candidate had won every prior election since 1988. In 2016, Donald Trump won the state by about 11,000 votes, a 0.23% margin. Basically, the state's voters were split evenly between Democrats and Republicans in 2016.

Like everyone else, Katey was glued to these 2016 presidential election results. But she also was paying attention to what was happening in elections in Michigan for the US House of Representatives and the state legislature. That November, Republicans won 9 US congressional seats in Michigan and Democrats only won 5. But if you look at the vote totals in congressional races across the state, you see that Republican candidates for the US House of Representatives won 48% of votes and Democratic US House candidates won 47% of votes—a 1% margin. Given it was an even split, why weren't the seats also evenly split, 7 and 7? Or at least 8 and 6?

Katey was also looking at the Michigan state legislature results. In the popular vote across all of the races in the Michigan House of Representatives, Republicans won 49.2% of the vote and Democrats won 49.1% of the vote.[267] Again, an almost exact split between the parties. Yet Republicans retained control of the lower house of the Michigan legislature by winning 63 seats compared to Democrats only winning 47 seats. There were about the same number of Democrat voters as there were Republican voters, but Democrats were packed into specific districts and thus won fewer seats. There were 7 districts that Democrats won by over 90% whereas there was no district that Republicans won by more than 75%.

These lopsided results, despite the even split on votes, is largely due to partisan gerrymandering. After the new census results were released in 2010, each state in the country had to do redistricting. In Michigan, like most other states, the responsibility for creating the maps for redistricting fell to the state legislature. At the time, the Republicans controlled the Michigan state legislature, so they were able to create maps that helped entrench their advantage. Their new maps were successful. In the 2012 elections using the new maps, Democrats won 54% of the popular vote but still lost the Michigan House of Representatives with only 51 seats compared to 59 seats for the Republicans.[268] This process of creating districts for partisan advantage—often in odd shapes or splitting communities in ways that do not make sense—is called partisan gerrymandering.

Twenty-seven-year-old Katey Fahey saw the 2016 results in her state and believed that the political system was unfair. The local news outlet *Bridge Michigan* told her story.[269] In the days after the 2016 election, she was scrolling her social media feeds and seeing a lot of anger being posted by friends and relatives. Fahey is from the westside of Michigan and had never been part of political organizing. But she knew she wanted to do something about the anger she felt and the unjust political system we were all a part of.

She wrote in a Facebook post: "I'd like to take on gerrymandering in Michigan. . . . If you're interested in doing this as well please let me know." Katie recognized that gerrymandering was a root cause of the seemingly unfair and antidemocratic outcome of 9 Republicans and 5 Democrats in the US House of Representatives and a Republican majority in the State House, despite near-even splits in the popular votes. She, like many other residents who believed in the concept of democracy, believed it would be more fair for the representatives to more accurately reflect the voters in the state.

The response to Katey's Facebook post was immediate, and she quickly created a Facebook group to gather people with energy around the issue. She eventually pulled together a phone call with about 50 volunteers who then subdivided into committees and started to get things done. They worked toward the goal of getting citizen-created district maps as a ballot initiative for the 2018 election. To do so, they needed to get hundreds of thousands of petition signatures by citizens, something that typically requires millions of dollars and the help of political professionals. Katey's all-volunteer team ended up getting 400,000 signatures well before the deadline—85,000 more signatures than was required by law.

Thanks to the efforts of Katey and her volunteers, Michigan voters were able to vote on a proposal in the November 2018 election. If passed, the proposal would establish a nonpartisan commission of citizens. The commission's task:

Establish new redistricting criteria including geographically compact and contiguous districts of equal population, reflecting Michigan's diverse population and communities of interest. Districts shall not provide disproportionate advantage to political parties or candidates.

This new law would, in effect, take power away from the partisan state legislature so that a nonpartisan commission of citizens could draw the maps in ways that did not create partisan advantages.

Despite Michigan's penchant for close election results, the 2018 proposal—Prop 2 as it was called—passed by 22 percentage points: 61% to 39%. In the years that followed, a citizen's redistricting commission was established, and new maps were drawn after the 2020 census. The 2022 elections were the first to use those new maps, and the results were dramatically different. In the November 2022 elections for US House delegation from Michigan, Democrats won 51% of the statewide vote and 7 seats while the Republicans won 48% of the vote and 6 seats. It was an even-ish popular vote with even-ish results for representation. In the Michigan House of Representatives, Democrats won 56 seats and 51% of the popular vote; Republicans won 54 seats and 49% of the popular vote.[270] The 2024 election results similarly resulted in somewhat even vote splits and division of seats between each party. The new maps helped to ensure that the proportion of representatives that a party earned in the State House matched the proportion of votes it received statewide.

Through the work of Katey and her volunteers, as well as residents getting out to vote, a root cause of inequity in Michigan's political system was eliminated and replaced with a more just and equitable system that can be more reflective of residents' opinions on the issues.

The work of Katey and her team is a prime example of those famous words attributed to Margaret Mead: "Never doubt that a small group of thoughtful, committed, citizens can change the world." So who is your small group? Who can you connect with? What is your local issue?

Katey's work also connects with the epigraph at the beginning of this chapter, which comes from the book *Viral Justice* by Ruha

Benjamin. This excellent book implores the "low-key scheming of everyday people." It doesn't always have to be a big hearing on Capitol Hill or a courtroom fight. It can start from a Facebook post, a text to a group chat, or a community event. Benjamin urges us to be inspired by, rather than fearful of, viruses. She writes:

What if, instead, we reimagined virality as something we might learn from? What if the virus is not something simply to be feared and eliminated, but a microscopic model of what it could look like to spread justice and joy in small but perceptible ways? Little by little, day by day, starting in our own backyards, let's identify our plots, get to the root cause of what's ailing us, accept our interconnectedness.[271]

Those smaller actions can start to have bigger impacts. Benjamin's book is inspiring and full of examples of "viral justice." It is all around us. Most of the rights that we hold dear or the policies that help us thrive are the result of the "low-key scheming of everyday people."

What are the things that we can do? What type of scheming can we do? These are questions that I get from my students and other audiences all the time. I teach them about the centuries of history in this country that have led to the vast inequities in the present day. The weight of that history hangs heavy in the classroom, but that history also includes example after example of everyday people scheming and fighting and collaborating to make the world a better place. It is easy to think that all is hopeless. But the reality is that there are things we can do. We can all play a role in planting seed for a more equitable and just future.

* * *

When my kids were a bit younger, a scene played on repeat in our household. Usually, we would finish up dinner and play with the kids for a little bit, and then my wife or I would notice the time and realize that we needed to initiate the "bedtime routine." This routine started around 6:45 or 7 p.m., and most nights we started with cleaning up the mess we had made during the day. Inevitably, I would say, "Alright everyone, let's straighten up the house!" My three young children would usually respond with groans, sometimes tears, and occasionally by throwing themselves on the ground (to give them credit, about once a month—with no scientific way to predict when—they would simply respond by cleaning up).

I almost always had to talk them out of their groans, tears, and tantrums. Over the years, I have realized that the strategy that works best is to break down the task into smaller pieces. "Straighten up the house" is simply too daunting, even for our relatively small ranch home. My kids' first response was usually to cry: "But that will take forever!"

What they needed from me was to break down the task into smaller pieces. "Kid 1, pick up the 24 small plastic fish that are scattered on the floor in the playroom." "Kid 2, take a towel and wipe up the water that someone dripped from the bath into the kitchen and then into their bedroom." "Kid 3, grab a washcloth and wipe up the chocolate (and hopefully not poop) fingerprint on the wall." The house is a mess, but really it is just a series of smaller tasks to get it tidy again.

This concept is equally true for my students. I give them an assignment to write a 10-page single-space grant proposal and tell them that they have the whole semester to write it. It seems extremely daunting until I break it up into eight small pieces that they will work on one by one throughout the semester. Then, each assignment becomes easier, and I receive fewer emails from stressed-out students who are overwhelmed by the task at hand. I work the same way. Writing this book only seemed feasible once I broke it down into a list of smaller tasks spread out over a year.

Transforming our society is like that. It is the mother of all tasks. It is actually a bit hard to think of a task that is bigger than that. So, we are going to need to break it down into smaller pieces to better understand how we might approach it. When I think about what we can do, I draw on some lessons that I have learned from my friend and colleague Dr. Whitney Peoples. Whitney is a dynamic powerhouse. She has taught me so many important lessons about how to put anti-racist values into practice, how to disrupt harmful hierarchies, and how to lead organizational change. Whitney and I first met when she had a role helping instructors at the University of Michigan adopt anti-racist teaching principles, one of Whitney's areas of expertise. She taught me that an anti-racist teacher needs to think about several dimensions of teaching, including *where* we teach, *how* we teach, and *what* we teach. (This idea is partially drawn from writing by Kyoko Kishimoto.[272]) Because I am a teacher, this guidance is very relevant to me. But, more broadly, those who are seeking to transform our society can take this guidance and use it more expansively. We must think about the following:

- *Where* we work for transformation
- *How* we approach transformation
- *What* we try to transform

* * *

In the subsequent chapters, we will start with *where we transform*, and break it down into a chapter on transforming ourselves and a chapter on transforming our communities, with concrete areas where we can focus our energies. Then, we will take a similar approach in discussing *how we approach transformation*, which entails building relationships and working in partnership, working for equity rather than equality, and using an anti-racist approach. Finally, we will move into *what we need to transform*, including redressing our history, changing democratic systems, shifting social norms, engaging in mutual aid, and disrupting power relations.

CHAPTER 10

Where We Transform, Ourselves

You must be the change you wish to see in the world.
—Mahatma Gandhi

Chicago-based artist Olly Costello has a piece of art that shows someone pulling up roots from inside themselves. The accompanying text says, "Uproot tendencies towards policing others that exist inside you."[273] The artwork asks us to disrupt and change how we think about our role in policing other people's behaviors because of the harms that policing can have on others. The message of "uprooting tendencies" within ourselves has broad applications when we think about transforming our society.

All of us have been affected by the narratives, values, and messaging that has been dominant in our society. The racism, sexism, homophobia, transphobia, and other systems of oppression and advantage are embedded in almost all aspects of life. No matter who we are, those narratives, values, and messages have shaped us. To transform our society, we need to start with the active personal work of recognizing those harmful ideas within us and uprooting those tendencies.

Have you ever listened in on elementary schoolkids talking with their friends on the playground? You will often hear them referring to "good guys" and "bad guys." It is a quick and easy shorthand to divide the world up in this way. Adults do this same thing. They will say, "He's a bad dude" or refer to people as "criminals" or "felons." Just take a look at a newspaper. People are frequently reduced to their worst action by being labeled as a tax cheat, murderer, or drug dealer. Our cognitive shortcuts lead us to place those folks in the "bad guy" category.

But what are we really saying when we label people in this way? It is true that there are some people who have done truly heinous things and have made *bad choices*. But most people who have harmed someone else—or support policies that harm others—have also been a supportive friend or caring parent at other moments in their life. And evidence shows that most perpetrators have previously been victims of harm.[274] It is simply not as easy as we would like to think to divide the world into good guys and bad guys. All of us have a history that is a mix of good behaviors and bad behaviors.

The "bad guy" framing reinforces our desire to treat people differently, put people in jail, or deprive them of opportunities and resources. If someone is a *bad guy*, then the logical solution is to somehow cut them off from society and keep them away from everyone. But what if a human merely made a *bad choice*? How we talk about and frame an issue will ultimately change how we think about solutions and public policies to address it. Transforming ourselves to see the humanity in everyone—even those who have made bad choices—is an important step in "uprooting tendencies within ourselves" that can harm others.

* * *

The insidious nature of systems of oppression and privilege is that they are held not just by the people in the advantaged position but also those who are harmed. It is no surprise to anyone that a man might hold patriarchal beliefs or a white person might believe in white supremacy. But it is not uncommon for women to uphold those patriarchal beliefs, and people of color can hold racist ideas or uphold white supremacy. This is sometimes called internalized oppression.

Poet Kyle "Guante" Tran Myhre wrote, "White Supremacy is not a shark, it is the water."[275] Unfortunately, it is something we are all swimming in. Patriarchy, ableism, and other systems also work like that. Until we truly see it and understand it, we will blindly be influenced by it. Like the story told by David Foster Wallace, we do not always recognize the water we are swimming in. The fish ask, "What's water?"

In Malcolm X's autobiography, he writes at length about the anti-Black racism he embodied and felt. He describes how he would conk his hair, a popular style for Black men in the 1940s because it straightened their hair and made it look more like a stereotypical white person's hair. Malcolm X wrote about the first of many times he conked his hair before he realized the internalized racism inherent in the practice:

> This was my first really big step toward self-degradation: when I endured all of that pain, literally burning my flesh to have it look like a white man's hair. I had joined that multitude of Negro men and women in America who are brainwashed into believing that the black people are "inferior"—and white people "superior"—that they will even violate and mutilate their God-created bodies to try to look "pretty" by white standards.[276]

Eventually, the "Black is Beautiful" movement helped to name some of the anti-Black racism present in beauty standards and galvanize Black people to embrace and value their natural features, including their hair. Malcolm X's example shows how racist cultural ideas can seep into every corner of society. He was uprooting the white supremacist beauty standards that lived within him.

Once we start digging in and taking a critical eye, we start to notice all the different tendencies we need to uproot in ourselves. Many of them have been described in previous sections of the book. We need to uproot the idea that we live in a meritocracy where the smartest and hardest-working people are the ones who rise to the top and are successful. We need to uproot the idea that competition for resources through capitalism provides the best conditions for everyone. We need to uproot the idea that humans are superior to nature and can simply use the natural world as an expendable resource. We need to uproot the idea that health care and other basic needs are commodities rather than human rights.

* * *

I am going to let you in on a secret that I didn't use to admit. In my field, people use a certain word—*praxis*—that is really important, but I did not fully understand its meaning for the longest time. If someone used the word in a conversation, I would just nod along and hope that context clues would help me keep up with the conversation. When it was written, I would just skip over it and move along. But then I finally *got* what it means, and it is a wonderful word!

Paolo Freire writes in *Pedagogy of the Oppressed* that praxis is "reflection and action directed at the structures to be transformed."[277] It is this cycle that is critically important for how we approach change work. People often are so eager to do what makes them feel like they made a difference that they skip straight to the action part. But, without critical self-reflection, we are likely to take action without fully recognizing our own role in the problem and the best strategies to pursue to make lasting change.

Nonprofits and businesses are littered with stories of people who took "action" to make change but actually contributed to the problem more than they helped solve it. Consider the Italian development organization that thought it could just teach Zambians how to farm but actually wasted everyone's time because—as the Zambians knew would happen—hippos ate all the crops.[278] Critical self-reflection cannot always prevent these types of errors, but it is a way to approach change-making in a more effective manner.

There are several strategies you can use to engage in self-reflection. In a post on Twitter that has since been deleted, activist Mariame Kaba outlines this practice:

Questions I regularly ask myself when I'm outraged about injustice:

1. *What resources exist so I can better educate myself?*
2. *Who's already doing work around this injustice?*
3. *Do I have the capacity to offer concrete support and help to them?*
4. *How can I be constructive?*[279]

These reflection questions are critically important to help ground any action. We all have a tendency to rush to action. When we are outraged, it feels good to take action immediately. Truly following the questions outlined by Kaba requires some effort. But, if the Italian aid organization had followed these questions, they might have ended up learning from local Zambians and partnering to take a much different action that would have led to better outcomes for Zambians.

Better educating yourself and finding out who is doing the work could take an afternoon or two, and even then, you are likely just scratching the surface. Nonetheless, these types of reflections—before taking action—can help you to take more meaningful action. This work is not always easy. But if we recognize our own connection to these harmful systems—whether it be as a beneficiary or a harmed person—and if we want to transform them, we need to take the time to be intentional about how we engage.

The concept of praxis suggests that we need to engage in a cycle of reflection, action, reflection, action, reflection, action, and so on. This concept reminds us that our reflection is never over, and neither is our action. They work in tandem to move us toward the future we want to live in.

* * *

Have you ever tried to change something in your life? If you are like me, your brain is always eager for the next thing that will make life easier or more efficient or happier. It might fall into the category of #LifeHack, or it might be a new technology. For example, do you know that beautiful tablet-slash-Kindle device that lets you take notes and then magically upload and turn them into digital form? In my weak moments, when Instagram smartly serves me up this advertisement, I tell myself that this technological product will *completely transform* my life. It will make me more organized, more on top of my commitments, less forgetful, a better husband and father, and a better human being. And I will look *so cool* holding it. Why on earth wouldn't I spend the hundreds of dollars to buy it if those are the outcomes?

Well, I need to be *thoughtful* about how I approach this predicament. I have identified some problems: I am an inconsistent notetaker; I take notes in all sorts of random places; and I rarely actually look back at my notes. Those habits make me forget to-dos and details, which makes me feel like I am dropping the ball on some of my commitments and relationships.

Would this miracle tablet solve *those* problems? How would ownership of this device solve my problem of being an inconsistent notetaker? How would it solve my problem of rarely looking back to my notes? Admittedly, it *might* help me have all my notes in the same place. But that will require me to be tethered to this product, which is something I have never been able to do with a simple notebook. At any given time, I might have four different notebooks that I take notes in, and often they are not actually with me, so I take notes on scrap pieces of paper or on my phone. As I write this paragraph, there are scattered post-its with random notes surrounding my computer.

So, what do I have to do? I have to know myself and reflect on what I really need to change. Will this technology change me and change my life? Likely not. What are my habits? What is my life like, and what is my history with new technologies? By asking these questions, I can draw better conclusions about what I can do to make an impact on this problem. If I focus on the problem and how I am connected to the problem, instead of skipping straight to solutions, then I can take better action and truly *transform my life.*

This same concept applies to how we think about transforming our world. You need to know yourself. It means critically reflecting on who you are as a person and what role you can play in a movement to transform our society. We need to ask ourselves how we are connected to an issue. Sometimes, the connection is and feels very personal. Other times it may seem tangential.

Given who I am and my identities, I do not have personal experience with much of the harms of our systems. Our harmful immigration policies create an underclass of undocumented Americans who labor without legal protections and under constant threat that they will be violently removed from their family here in the United States. I do not directly experience those harms. Given my work with immigrant communities in the United States, I have friends who do experience those harms, and it tears me up inside to think about how they have to navigate life in our society. But just because I don't experience those harms does not mean that I am not connected to them.

My family enjoys inexpensive supermarket fruit picked by undocumented farmworkers. I accumulate money in my bank account in other ways because of the low-wage underclass that this immigration system has created. The companies that I interact with use this low-wage labor force to clean their offices, work their factories, and harvest their farms. That great deal that I got from the restaurant down the street and from my cell phone company is partially built on the oppressive immigration policies that our country employs.

Some of you may hold a mix of advantages and disadvantages or more squarely hold identities that are being oppressed in this country. If you are thriving, you are doing so despite monumental barriers that have been placed in front of you by the systems and institutions in this country. If you are more directly harmed by a system, your role in changing it might look different than other peoples.

Understanding yourself and your position is critically important for seeing what your role might be for changing those very systems and institutions. There is a famous line attributed to Lilla Watson, an Indigenous Australian artist, activist, and academic: "If you have come here to help me you are wasting your time, but if you have come because your liberation is bound up with mine, then let us work together."

The first part of the quote is easy enough. People do not want to feel like they are a charity case: "If you have come here to help me you are wasting your time." If you approach this work of transforming our society solely from the perspective of trying to help people who are less advantaged, you are not seeing the whole picture. This isn't only about helping folks who are marginalized; this is about the entire system being bad for all of us. Is it worse for some more than others? Absolutely. But we need to reflect on how our "liberation is bound up with" one another. How am I—someone with many advantages in one of the wealthiest countries in the history of the world—not liberated? This is something I have struggled to understand. But when I delved deeper into who I was and how I was connected to the inequities in our society, I started to understand it better.

How am I not liberated? Because so many essentials in my life are tied to the exploitation of others and our planet. My ability to feed my family, enjoy leisurely weekends, travel, live in a beautiful home with ample space for my family, and frankly, to have the time and space to write this very book, it is all tied to underpaid workers and the exploitation of resources from our planet. Ideally, we would live in a society where everyone would have the same opportunities and resources as me, but unfortunately, the current structure of our society makes some of these things out of reach for many people.

Why did I hit the jackpot? Largely, by accident of my birth. Sure, I didn't screw it up along the way. I didn't flee from the educational path set in front of me, and I was able to grab the opportunities placed easily in front of me. Not everyone is able to do that, and it takes effort to stay the course, but the benefits are great. Many others have to put in so much more effort to fight to carve that path and opportunities for themselves.

A lot of people do not realize that their liberation *is bound up*. They are living life, and they are happy. And that is a joyful thing. But they have not critically examined the ways that their happy and joyful life is possible because of the exploitation of others and our planet. And they have not imagined a world where no one is exploited. But, once you let yourself see the world for what it is, rather than what you want it to be, you can see the ways in which your liberation is bound up with others.

Part of doing this work to know yourself and how you are connected to an issue is to see how you are *bound up* with the people who are most affected by the issue. If you are talking about the problem of incarceration, how are you bound up with that if you are not incarcerated yourself? If you are talking about the problem of human rights abuses against undocumented workers, how are you bound up with that if you are not an un-documented worker? If you are talking about the murder of trans women, how are you bound up with that problem if you are not a trans woman? We are all tied in certain ways to the harms plaguing our society. Recognizing and clearly articulating this fact can help you to identify the ways you can start to undo those problems in our society.

*   *   *

Working toward a better future requires us to return to the idea of seven generations. What we do today is not for ourselves but rather our great-great-great-great-great grandchildren. What seeds can we plant today that our descendants can reap?

We have to remind ourselves that our ancestors planted seeds for us. Think about the people fighting for the abolition of chat-tel slavery. Some of those people were not passionate about merely the abolition of slavery; they wanted Black people in America to *thrive*. Abolishing slavery was just a big step among many steps that were needed to allow Black people to thrive. In the present day, there are many Black people that are thriving in ways that their ancestors could not even imagine. That thriv-ing would not have been possible without the movements to abolish slavery, repeal Jim Crow laws, promote Black pride, en-shrine civil rights protections in the law, and fight to make Black Lives Matter. Of course, as this book has highlighted, there are many ways that Black Americans—and other marginalized groups—are prevented from thriving or are thriving despite the numerous disadvantages they face. What are we doing to ensure that the people living seven generations from now can all thrive and live in a world that is equitable and just?

Melissa Creary is a member of the faculty at the University of Michigan School of Public Health. She is a deep thinker, scholar, and activist on issues related to health equity and how we embed greater equity into our policies. She also is a Black woman living with sickle cell disease who has experienced firsthand how our systems, especially our health care system, can exclude or discriminate.[280] Dr. Creary introduced the concept of "bounded justice."[281] It has completely changed how many scholars, practitioners, and activists think about working toward equity and justice in our society. Bounded justice helps us to understand that deeply entrenched structural racism will undercut any of our efforts at equity and justice. Simply put, we are not going to get to equity with our first attempt. The policy solution being proposed will not get us to justice. In that sense, we are "bounded" by our history and the systems we have in place. Even so, there is hope within this concept. People and institutions can expect these failures and plan for them. They can view these setbacks as part of the journey toward equity. Part of the lesson of bounded justice is that we must be resilient in our fight for equity and justice. We must view it as long-term work that lasts well beyond our lifetimes.

Michelle Alexander has written powerfully in the book *The New Jim Crow* about how structural racism has shape-shifted in this country from chattel slavery to Jim Crow segregation to mass incarceration.[258] Each time there was a success (e.g., abolishing slavery, passing civil rights legislation), there was a backlash. Two steps forward and one step back. Bounded justice allows us to see that the Civil Rights Act and other legislation of the 1960s was not going to fully provide the justice that people wanted. Its success would be undercut and more efforts would still be needed, and will continue to be needed, to get closer to justice.

As an example, the Fair Housing Act of 1968 included a provision that required action be taken to undo segregation and unequal opportunity.[282] This provision to affirmatively further fair housing was a huge legislative win in 1968 after decades of racist policies that created racially segregated neighborhoods with vastly different levels of investment and resources. It *would have been* a big win, but the presidential administrations that run the federal government, including the Department of Housing and Urban Development (HUD), declined to enforce that particular provision of the Fair Housing Act.

Nikole Hannah-Jones documented this important history in a ProPublica investigation titled "Living Apart: How the Government Betrayed a Landmark Civil Rights Law."[283] Her reporting showed that President Richard Nixon's HUD secretary tried to follow the Affirmatively Furthering Fair Housing (AFFH) provision by denying funding for federal projects within cities that were allowing racial segregation. But then white southerners and northern suburbanites complained to Nixon and he put a stop to it, thus ending any attempt at enforcement of the provision. Subsequent presidential administrations, both Republican and Democrats, failed to enforce the provision. It wasn't until late in the President Barack Obama's administration, in 2015, that HUD made and implemented a plan for enforcing the provision. The new AFFH rule was subsequently removed by Donald Trump's administration in 2020 and then reinstated again in 2021 under President Joseph Biden. The second Trump Administration quickly removed all mention of AFFH from HUD websites. Forward progress followed by backsliding.

One of the most important takeaways from the concept of bounded justice is that we need to be ready to fail and adapt and fail again and adapt. We cannot make a plan, execute, and think we are done. The work of equity and justice is long-term work. We have to think of it as a marathon or perhaps an ultramarathon rather than a sprint. The lyricist Brett Dennan wrote, *"I'm planting trees I'll never climb."* That is the mindset we need to bring to our work. We may not be the beneficiaries of the work we are doing today.

* * *

I have some experience shifting from shorter distances to long distances. My running life started when I was about 11 years old, when my dad told my sisters and me that we all had to "train" for an upcoming hiking trip in Colorado by running one mile around our neighborhood. After that, I started running one or two miles at a time to train for my high school soccer team and then developed a habit of running two or three miles a few times a week in college as part of staying healthy. Once my soon-to-be wife convinced me to start running longer distances, it was a completely different experience. I soon started training for a half-marathon, then a full marathon. Several years later, I completed a 40-mile run as a part of a race in the North Carolina mountains. I got hooked and, each year, I try to complete a few long-distance races and go on many long training runs to prepare.

I have had to shift my mindset completely in order to finish these longer-distance runs, similar to the way we need to shift our perspective when thinking about our work of making a better world. When running shorter distances, I would be thinking about the finish line from the start. "Almost done," I would tell myself. In contrast, once I started running marathons, I had to learn to break up the run into much shorter distances. The whole time, I know what my end goal is and how far the finish line is, but I am working toward mini goals along the way. If I just started the race and focused only on the finish line, I would likely lose my motivation.

The other thing I have learned from long-distance running is that in any given race, you will get discouraged several times, so you need the resilience to keep going. Perhaps you realize that you aren't going to make your time goal, or perhaps your leg is cramping up, or you just came upon a hill that completely wiped the energy you had left. This is the moment when the wind comes out of your sails. A voice creeps in and says, "You should just pull out of the race," or "It's fine—just walk the rest of the way." The length of the race makes you feel hopeless in these moments. *If I'm feeling this way at mile 14, how am I going to get all the way until mile 26? Is it worth it?* Just like the resilience highlighted by the bounded justice theory, these moments of discouragement are exactly when you need to use all your available resources to pick yourself back up and keep going.

For me, in those moments, I use several strategies. Sometimes I turn to repeating mantras. One trail marathon through the woods of southern Michigan had me feeling hopeless after what seemed like a roller coaster of endless hills. I started to whisper "you've got this" with every exhaled breath to remind myself of my own strength. In a different trail marathon, I envisioned my beloved dog and running companion by my side, pulling me along with his leash. In city road races, I try to find spectators who can cheer for me or slap my hand to give me a bit of an emotional boost. Other times, I take a short walk-break to eat something for some extra energy. I have learned to be resilient in these moments because I know that meeting my goal depends on me finding a way through the challenges. I have grown to *expect* the challenges. I know they are coming, so I have my toolkit of strategies ready to tackle them. It doesn't mean they aren't still a huge challenge, but it means I know I can and should keep going.

The other thing I have learned from these long-distance races is that support and teamwork is absolutely essential. To this day, I have never run a marathon distance or longer by myself. It is always done within a community of runners who are also tackling the same goal at the same time. This community of runners is a beautiful thing. We give each other words of encouragement as we pass each other and check on each other mid-race if someone seems injured or struggling. The power of community provides some of the strength to face the challenge. Beyond the other runners, every one of us is supported by many. My family supports me to train and often comes to cheer me on. Volunteers come to the race to set up aid stations with food, water, and first aid. Neighbors come out and cheer; they bring inspiration and funny signs. It would be infinitely harder to run these distances without all of this support in place.

When we are thinking about the long-term nature of transforming our society, we have to approach it like an ultramarathon. Know that there is an end goal but focus on the shorter markers of progress. Find your community of fellow runners. Find your support crew. Adopt a mindset that is expecting challenges, and plan ahead for your strategies to overcome them. Hold on to the faith and continue moving forward.

* * *

Working on ourselves is a fundamental if we want to contribute to making a better world possible. After embarking on the work within ourselves, we can think about transforming our communities.

CHAPTER 11

Where We Transform, Our Communities

Nothing will work, unless you do.
—Maya Angelou

Recall that in the book *Viral Justice* by Ruha Benjamin, the author invites the reader to take action by finding their own plot and tending it.[271] She suggests that we care for and create change within our plots to create the beautiful and bountiful garden we desire. This perspective is key to creating the societal changes we need to transform at the root. People with privilege often have a tendency to locate problems within other people or communities and envision working to fix *those* problems. But what if we shift that lens and begin to think about transformation within our own communities, organizations, and institutions? What role do each of these play in contributing to the problems and solutions within our society? When we think about where we can focus our energy, it is often right under our nose.

* * *

As a high school student, I had a vague interest in politics and government, and my school offered students the opportunity to take a day off to shadow someone who had a career that interested them. I was planning on going to college and majoring in political science. I didn't live in Washington, D.C., and the state capital was three hours away, so local government was the closest thing I could think of that might be relevant to my career interests. I shadowed our city administrator in the suburban town of 35,000 where I lived. I vividly remember sitting in a bland conference room with beige walls and an uninteresting table while a group of middle-aged people wearing khakis discussed what type of decorations our town would have on its streetlights. I was supremely uninterested. This is what policymaking and local government looked like? Count me out, thought my 18-year-old self.

Fast-forward to today, where I realize just how critical and important local government is. All right, maybe not the decisions about streetlights and the other mundane things that make a city function. But I came to realize that housing policy and zoning (a very unsexy but important policy topic) were controlled by local government officials. Much of the policing and jails that local residents interact with were under the purview of local government. Resources for homeless individuals, funding and curriculum for schools, and budgets for public parks and libraries were all decided by local governing bodies. Sometimes, local officials had to make mundane decisions, too, but if I cared about issues of equity and justice, then starting locally made a lot of sense.

I used to be someone who was caught up in the national news cycles. I was interested in the president's actions, federal policy proposals, and political fights. Many of those policies had so many stakeholders involved in the process that it was hard to know where I fit in. I did not have a good sense of where I could plug in. National politics is still crucially important, but often the best way to plug into issues that you care about is by engaging with your own local community.

One key distinction here is that focusing on your own community does not mean that you ignore issues outside your community. This is especially true if you are from a well-resourced community. If we only invest our time and resources in our own community, we may exacerbate inequities. But acting locally is also a way to change how your community relates or contributes to those inequities. Thinking about local schools is a great example.

Not only are school districts in wealthier communities better funded by local property taxes, the Parent-Teacher Organizations (PTOs) in those communities are also wealthier since the parents have more to donate and give. It creates a situation where some school districts have all their basic needs—and much more—met while other districts are lacking key resources to be able to provide a thorough education to their students. So, if people in well-resourced communities simply focus on their own community, does that mean you have to just add to the inequities?

The key is to work on our own communities and think about how our own community contributes to this dynamic of inequity. There are some things that you could advocate for in your own community that would have spillover benefits for other communities that are lacking in resources. For example, you could advocate that your PTO donates half of the proceeds from its yearly fundraiser to a school district with fewer resources. Even better, you could leverage the power that your wealthy community holds to advocate for a fairer distribution of education funding in your state. After all, it is wealthy communities that are typically those that argue against this type of reform. This would mean working locally in your own community to convince wealthy or powerful actors to join your efforts to make educational funding more equitable. Do not fall into the trap that all local advocacy is good advocacy; it needs to take a critical lens to inequities and contribute to reducing inequities.

* * *

In your own community, you likely have relationships to build on and local knowledge of how things get done. You have the capacity to bring people together and mobilize them. At its simplest level, it is inviting one or two friends for coffee and saying, "There is an issue that's been on my mind. Can we take a moment to talk a bit about how we make an impact?" That issue could be about electing a local candidate who is advocating for changes or a new initiative in your neighborhood. Find a friend, start learning more, and then take action together.

Thus far, I have been using the word *community* without putting many parameters on it. This is intentional since your community can be however you define it. You might think very specifically of your neighborhood or the city or town where you live, or perhaps you have a wider perspective that includes your entire state. Or, you might think about your faith community or ethnic community. You might even think about the online community of folks you are connected with through social media or an affinity group you are a part of. The point is that your actions do not need to be geographically located; rather, you need to work on change within the network of people you are already connected to. If you are drawn to change-making in other communities that are not your own, spend the time to first build relationships in those spaces and be guided by folks who are rooted in that group. Any change is built on a foundation of relationships and connections; that is your starting place.

* * *

Beyond our loved ones and our communities, our sphere of possible influence also extends into the institutions and organizations that we are a part of. What are the institutions you are closely connected to?

When I ask myself this question, I think about where I work: the University of Michigan, the School of Public Health, and the specific department I work within. I also think about groups I have been a part of, including the Michigan chapter of Public Health Awakened and the Coalition for Reenvisioning Our

Safety. I am also a member of the American Public Health Association and a parent at my kid's elementary school. There are many other organizations and institutions that I am connected to in different ways, but these are some of the core ones and spaces where I can focus some of my energy for change.

There are two ways to think about our work with organizations and institutions that we are connected to. First, how can I change this particular institution to shift toward a root cause perspective and help reduce inequities? In this way, we are thinking about exercising our power within these spaces to shift organizational policies or practices. Second, we can think about how we direct the power and energy of these institutions and organizations toward a particular issue or policy that is external to the organization. I will give an example of each of these cases.

Internal institutional change is about changing the policies and practices of the institutions or organizations we are a part of. At the University of Michigan School of Public Health, applicants previously had to take the Graduate Record Exam (GRE) to be admitted to our graduate programs. In public health, the masters of public health degree is one of the most prominent required degrees to get many mid-level jobs, so the GRE can be a gateway into the next level of the profession.

There has been a movement to drop GRE requirements from graduate admissions because (a) the test has been shown to discriminate based on race and gender and (b) it was hard to take the GRE during the COVID-19 pandemic.[284,285] One of the (many) root causes of why the public health profession was not as diverse as it should be is because students of color and from other marginalized backgrounds were disadvantaged when they took the test. Repeated studies showed that the test was not a good predictor of graduate success and was more a marker of race and class.[286,287] So people who were poor or from non-

European heritage scored lower because of how the test was created.

At the School of Public Health, removing the GRE test as a requirement would cost zero dollars. So, it was not a matter of convincing administrators to fork over money for a new program, but we needed to convince decision-makers that the school would not be harmed by such a change. As an elite university, there was concern that the removal of the GRE requirement could reduce the quality of our students if there was no standardized way to assess applicants. That is a whole other ball of wax to unpack, but the research showed that this change would not decrease the quality of students. Changing the GRE requirement at the institutional level had the potential to change our institution and make it more accessible to a range of diverse students. That would have downstream impacts on the type of people who would be part of the public health profession. And it would affect the types of people who had access to a masters of public health education from the University of Michigan, which could very likely lead to well-paying jobs in government, nonprofits, or industry for people who had historically been locked out of those opportunities.

As this issue started to be discussed at my institution, I thought about what role I could play in changing the policy. I first sought out information on how this decision would be made. I recognized it would be useful to share concerns about the GRE with key decision-makers across the school, especially people in roles closely connected to admissions. I did not hold much formal power or close relationships with these decision-makers, but I was part of a few groups that I thought I could mobilize around this issue. I brought up the issue with our diversity, equity, and inclusion committee that included students, faculty, and staff, and we brainstormed how we might communicate our concerns. The students agreed that they would talk to other students about sharing their concerns about the GRE with decision-makers. We also agreed that the faculty would reach out to our peers across the school to share some of our concerns about the GRE and share our opinion that dropping the GRE was the most equitable option for the school. If our colleagues shared our concerns, we asked them if they would be willing to bring up the concerns at their next faculty meeting or directly with decision-makers.

Through this process, we also learned a bit more about which decision-makers were resistant and which were already on board with the shift in policy. This way we could focus our energy a bit more. Our group was certainly not the only actor pushing for change in the school, but our efforts added to the collective energy around changing the policy.

After these efforts, the school announced that it would undertake a yearlong pilot during which time GRE scores would not be required for admission. Eventually, after that pilot period, there was a permanent removal of the GRE requirement. The GRE policy is an example of a policy that produces inequities and how an organized group within an institution can advocate for change.

*   *   *

The other way to think about transformation within institutions concerns how to harness the power of your organization or institution to instigate change outside the organization. One of the best examples that I have seen was led by a group of public health students and workers who were helping the 25,000-member American Public Health Association (APHA) promote public safety. They did so through recommendations to reduce police violence in society and by advocating for more life-affirming and safety-promoting social services.

The End Police Violence Collective has its origins at San Francisco State University, where a few students were writing about how police violence negatively affects the health of Black communities.[289] Eventually, those folks linked up with students at the University of Illinois at Chicago and set a goal of writing an APHA policy statement—"Addressing Law Enforcement Violence as a Public Health Issue"—that would be passed by the APHA executive committee. These were people who were part of APHA, although they were relatively junior members without any position of authority, yet they wanted to influence the organization to take a stand on this issue.

At the time, policy statements needed to be voted on and, if passed, were considered to be the official position of the APHA. Given that APHA is the leading public health advocacy body in the United States and that policy statements "provide the evidence base for legislative and regulatory recommendations,"[288] passing a policy statement helped to put the weight of the APHA behind an issue.

The group's proposed policy statement on "Addressing Law Enforcement Violence as a Public Health Issue" failed to pass at the 2017 APHA annual meeting. It only received 45% of the vote from the executive committee. Organizers were disappointed but did not give up. They knew they had work to do over the coming year to ensure that the policy statement would pass in 2018. They worked more closely with existing APHA members who held leadership positions to educate and persuade them to support the policy statement. They also did work to bring influential public health leaders on board with the policy statement.

At the 2018 APHA annual conference in San Diego, I attended a rally organized by the End Police Violence Collective in support of a policy statement on police violence as a public health issue.[289] Dr. Camara Phyllis Jones, renowned scholar of racism and well-respected past president of the APHA, was at the front of the march with other supporters holding a large banner that read "Health Equity Now: End Police Violence." The rally was organized to demonstrate a broad show of support for the passage of the policy statement.

It worked. The APHA executive committee met in the hours after the rally and voted on the policy statement. It passed 87% to 13%. This meant that the policy statement would now be posted on the APHA website and would inform the organization's advocacy actions. The final policy statement was well researched and made some key policy recommendations for federal, state, tribal, and local authorities.

What does the passage of such a policy statement do? Police violence is often viewed as a hot-button topic. But this policy statement lends support for public health professors like myself to discuss police violence as part of our public health curriculum. After all, the largest society of public health professionals has declared it a public health issue. The policy statement also means that studying police violence as a public health issue becomes a much more valid position, and public health researchers can refer to the statement in their grant proposals. It means that public health officials can and should play a role in policies related to public safety within their communities rather than ceding that territory solely to law enforcement officials. It provided cover for public health workers to talk about and take action on the issue.

In 2020, with protests erupting nationwide following the murder of George Floyd, the *New York Times* described police violence as having "become a major public health and civil rights issue."[290] Without the passage of that APHA policy statement, I do not think the paper would have described police violence as a "major public health issue."

So, what does this broader recognition of policing as a public health issue gain us? It means that some people will look at the issue differently. It means that the general public will not see police violence as only an issue of the criminal legal system that needs to be solved by lawyers and judges and police officers, but rather one that needs to be considered through a lens of prevention and equity that public health brings. It means that public health professionals—those who are trained in community engagement and developing programs aimed at prevention—will be better able to have a seat at the table in pushing for solutions. You personally may or may not agree that public health professionals should have a seat at the table, but the point is that the advocacy efforts to pass the APHA policy statement (among other organizing efforts by the public health community) have helped to shape the terms of this issue in the field of public health and, more importantly, in the public's eye.

This is the story of organizing *within* to put the weight of your institution or community behind a particular issue. What institutions or groups are you a part of? Have they gotten involved in important social change issues? How could you work with allies within your PTO, your workplace, or your church to help them take action on an issue important to you?

CHAPTER 12

How We Transform

We urgently need to bring to our communities the limitless capacity to love, serve, and create for and with each other. We urgently need to bring the neighbor back into our hoods, not only in our inner cities but also in our suburbs, our gated communities, on Main Street and Wall Street, and on Ivy League campuses.

—Grace Lee Boggs, *The Next American Revolution: Sustainable Activism for the Twenty-First Century*

We need to be very intentional and thoughtful about *how* we approach transformation. We can be guided by certain concepts and principles that set up the conditions for impactful work. This chapter digs into several of these ideas—namely, building relationships and working in partnership, working for equity rather than equality, and using an anti-racist approach—that can guide us in *how we approach transformation.*

* * *

When I joined the Peace Corps, it was a 27-month commitment. Three months of training would be followed by two years of service. In January 2007, I joined a group of 19 other volunteers focused on community health in Nicaragua. When we arrived in the country, we were divided into groups of four, and each group was sent to a different village within a cluster of towns in the southern part of the country. We each lived with a family so that we could practice our Spanish and better learn the culture and customs of our new home. Each group of four had a Nicaraguan-language teacher come visit our new homes several days a week to help us improve our Spanish. The other days we all came together for training on how to approach working within a community.

As I have gotten to know more former Peace Corps volunteers over the years, a common thread is that wherever they were in the world, they learned the importance of starting with relationships first. Whether it was drinking pinolillo in a rocking chair, chatting under a baobab tree, or sharing tea and a snack, a key part of the ethos of any Peace Corps volunteer was to take time to build relationships before diving into any work.

That relationship-building was the foundation for working in partnership with communities. The training we received during those three months drilled into us that our job was *not* to solve the community's problems. Our job was to listen. Our job was to lend support where we could. Our job was to work *hombro-a-hombro* (shoulder to shoulder) with members of our community to work on the issues they had identified as a priority.

So what did this look like, practically speaking? After the three-month training period was over, I was assigned to live in Corinto, a port town of about 20,000 set along the northern Pacific coast in the hottest region of the country. One day in late March 2007, I was dropped off by a Peace Corps staff member with my large duffel bag at a chaotic outdoor bus station and market in Nicaragua's capital city. There were no signs telling you where to go or indicating destinations; instead, the drivers or their assistants would roam the outdoor bus station shouting out their destination, hoping to scurry you to their bus. That day, I was listening for a sweaty young man shouting, "Corinto-Corinto-Corinto-Corinto-CORINTOOOOOOOOOOO." But of course, every other driver saw a lost-looking gringo and thought they might be able to convince me to go to with them to their destination. I swatted away those other offers, confident that I already had committed to enough adventure for one day. I eventually heard the call I was listening for and was guided toward a decades-old yellow school bus with big colorful letters painted above the windshield: "C-O-R-I-N-T-O." I lugged my big duffel bag with all my possessions onto the bus and would be on my way.

Thankfully, I arrived and found my way to the family in Corinto that I would be living with for the first few months and to the health clinic where I would be working with one of their community-health outreach workers. Our training told us that we should spend our first six months building relationships, listening to community members, and learning about our new community.

The folks in my new town were a bit surprised by this approach. They were used to gringos coming in thinking they had the "answers," executing a project, and leaving. This was a common occurrence. Church groups and businesses from the United States came, carried out a project, and left. Other international nonprofit or government organizations also came in to build some piece of infrastructure or deliver a program. When I would meet people, they always asked what I was there to do. When I told them, "I'm not sure yet," and offered to help them with anything they needed, their look of confusion made me feel that I was wasting everyone's time.

But in those first few months, I was able to connect with people and offer a hand with the projects they were working on. Sometimes, I would merely help them file papers at the clinic, prepare materials for a health education session, or take my bike to run an errand for someone. In one of the most interesting adventures in those early days, I tagged along and carried a small cooler on a door-to-door vaccination campaign, helping to ensure that all the town's kids were vaccinated against basic diseases. I would go with the team to some small remote islands off the coast, where a few hundred people lived with no roads, running water, or electricity. We pulled our tiny boat up along the beach and trudged along small paths that would eventually lead to a different cluster of shacks. Was I an essential part of the team? Not really, but they did appreciate the help lugging equipment. And more important, we had a lot of time to get to know each other. I got to visit almost every family in town and learned more about my new colleagues' jobs, their families, and their lives.

In those initial months, I would quickly adopt the local customs of never leaving home without my sweat rag to wipe my brow and occasionally "turning on the air conditioning" (as my new neighbors called it) by pulling up my shirt to expose my midriff to get some small amount of relief from the heat. But I also learned more important aspects of daily life in Corinto, such as the way that religion influenced people or the existing opportunities (or lack of) for paid work. I had to know the community before I could truly partner with them.

Eventually, as our relationships built up over time, people would come to me asking for partnership in an upcoming project, and I started feeling comfortable raising potential project ideas in our conversations. For example, Xiomara and I discussed how there was almost no health-related outreach for men in the community. We ended up co-creating a health education program for young men in the town, including a tournament at a popular billiards hall. In between tournament rounds, players had to listen to a short *charla* about health and then shout out answers to trivia questions. When I first joined the community, I had no knowledge of this service gap, and I could have never carried out a successful program on my own. The partnership and listening was key to being able to have an impact. When we think about *how* we transform our society, we need to start with building strong, trusting relationships. This helps to enable more effective partnerships for action.

* * *

I work in a job where productivity is always on my mind. There is always one more journal article to write, grant to submit, or student group to speak with. Having lunch with a colleague *feels* like it would simply be taking time away from *producing* something else. Even in some activist spaces that I have been in, we struggle to make time for simply hanging out and getting to know one another. But this attitude will not necessarily lead us to the future we need. Strong relationships will actually make the work of change possible.

My good friend teases me that I am always planning happy hours. "Happy hour" is our code word for anything that prioritizes being social and building relationships over just getting the work done. A meeting about a grant proposal? Not happy hour. Grabbing coffee with a few colleagues to chat generally about work life? Definitely a happy hour. It's true. I do have an affinity for planning these types of "happy hours." I have a bit of a history of planning social events, especially when I am in new spaces. I planned a true happy hour with beer and wine for fellow graduate students when I was a new graduate student at the University of North Carolina. I planned a meet-and-greet for junior faculty at my current workplace. I planned a playground meet-up for families in my neighborhood. Beyond these groups, I try to reach out to individuals and connect. Sometimes they are colleagues; sometimes they are folks who work at organizations that I partner with. Maybe my friend is right to tease me—it's an addiction.

But I have this desire to *know* the people in my life. I am deeply unsatisfied living in a neighborhood where I only wave "hi" to neighbors and then we all go about our day. I do not like workspaces where people show up to work and don't get past pleasantries. There are too many people in my office where the deepest interaction takes place in the hallways while we are rushing off to some meeting or other place. It goes like this:

Hey, how's everything going?
Oh, it's busy. I'm looking forward to this [week, month, semester] ending. How are you doing?
Same! I just keep waiting for it to let up.
Well, good luck! Hope things slow down for you.
Thanks. You, too!
Well, it was great to run into you.
You, too! Have a good one.
Bye!

It is fine to have some neighbors, some collaborators, and some colleagues who are surface-level acquaintances. We cannot have deep, meaningful relationships with every single person in our social network. The problem is that we infrequently create space to allow our relationships to go deeper than surface level.

I have one strategy that I like to use for going deeper than surface level, and it is one I draw from my research. It is similar to how community organizers do "relational organizing" with one-on-one meetings.[291] I often do qualitative research, which means that I conduct open-ended interviews with people. I have a specific population that I am focusing on (e.g., immigrants living in Detroit) and a specific research question (e.g., what are the barriers and facilitators to receiving adequate health care for this population?). Then, I recruit people to the study that fit the criteria, and I sit down with them and ask open-ended questions to gain insights that will help answer my research question. This is called a qualitative in-depth interview, and this type of approach can be wonderful for truly getting to know someone.

There are a few features of this type of interview that are especially helpful in delving deeper with someone. First, you have a set goal in mind. For me, the goal is to answer the research question, but the goal could be anything, such as "understand this person's values" or "understand more about this person's family and upbringing." You have planned some questions in advance (an interview guide) but are flexible to allow the conversation to take shape spontaneously. You also are focused on asking "probing questions" that allow the conversation to go deeper than it otherwise might. Often, the simplest probing question is either silence—the other person often fills the silence with more sharing—or simply asking, "Can you say more about that?"

The beauty of this type of conversation is that there is no expectation of a back-and-forth. One person is the focal point. They do not have to worry about talking too much and oversharing because that is what they are supposed to do! And the other person can truly listen because they are not worried about what they are supposed to say next. They can actually focus on what the person says. If you are using this strategy for relationship-building rather than for research, it would make sense to have two different sessions. This way, during one occasion, one person asks the questions, and then the next time, the other person asks the questions.

Deepening relationships in this way helps connect us to other people. It not only allows us to appreciate the diversity of the human experience, but it also helps us work together. When we understand someone's history, motivations, joys, and frustrations, we can work together more effectively for the long term. Relationships make open and honest communication possible in a way that surface-level connections do not allow. These networks of trusting relationships are one approach to how we transform. Next, we'll look at an equity approach.

* * *

When COVID-19 was ripping across the United States in the early days of the pandemic, Black and Hispanic Americans were being hit harder than other groups.[292] Eventually, effective vaccines were available in limited quantities. There were serious debates about who should have priority for accessing these vaccines. Most people agreed that health care workers on the front lines should be among the first to access the vaccines. In addition, most agreed that folks who were elderly should also be prioritized. But what about the racial groups that were hardest hit? Should they be able to have priority access? This question got at the heart of equity versus equality.

Equal distribution of vaccines would mean that vaccines would be available to every resident in an equal manner. This might look like a vaccine lottery—no group is a priority, and all people have an equal chance of getting early access to vaccines. In contrast, *equitable* distribution of vaccines would be distributing limited vaccines based on need, with certain groups being given early access. In the United States, we did see equitable distribution of vaccines on some dimensions of need, including the risk for complications from COVID (e.g., age or medical conditions) and the risk of exposure for frontline workers. But most places stopped short of giving priority for certain racial groups that had the most deaths.

You may be well aware of the cartoon illustrating the difference between equality and equity.[293] In the drawing labeled "equality," there are three spectators at a baseball game that are behind a wooden outfield fence that you cannot see through. The three individuals appear to be an adult, an adolescent, and a young child, and each of them is standing on an equal-sized crate to help them see over the fence. With the aid of the crate, the adult is easily able to see the field and is resting his hands on the top of the fence. The adolescent, who is shorter than the adult, can also see over the fence to have a clear view of the field. The crate makes them tall enough to have their shoulders, neck, and head above the fence. The young child is shorter than the adolescent, and the wooden crate does not help enough for them to see over the fence. So the child stands there with their hands at their side, staring straight at the wooden fence, without any view of the baseball field. This is the visual representation of equality: everyone gets the same resource—a crate—without regard to what each individual needs.

Next to the drawing of equality is a drawing representing the concept of equity. It is the same people, same fence, and same baseball game. This time, however, the three crates are distributed differently. Instead of each person getting one crate, the shortest person gets two crates, the medium-sized person gets one crate, and the tallest person gets no crate. With that assistance, the fence hits each of them at about shoulder height, and they can each comfortably see the action of the game. It is not hard to understand which one is a better outcome.

Some artists have done additional riffs on this famous image to help represent the concept of *justice*. If equality and equity are about distributing resources to overcome barriers, justice is about removing barriers altogether. In a view of justice in the world, the three spectators are viewing the game without a fence at all or through a chain-link fence that all can see through. In other words, the resources are focused on removing the barrier rather than trying to create a workaround solution.

When we think about transforming our society, it is critical to consider both the principles of equity and justice. With the goal of equal opportunity, we are likely going to have to distribute resources *equitably* rather than *equally*. When we think about high school education, some kids are going to need many more resources to catch up to kids who have had advantages. When we think about providing health care, we need to consider who has the most need and provide those extra supports and resources. As we think about making change in our communities and institutions, using an equity lens can help us to ensure that resources are distributed according to need instead of always defaulting to equal distribution.

When thinking about equity versus equality, it is important to take into account the distribution of resources that are considered a fundamental human right. A society may decide to distribute resources that are basic human rights *equally* across society. Falling into this category are education, health care, or basic income. There is a basic minimum standard that everyone should receive. This is the rationale behind the universal basic income proposals that are gaining traction.[294,295] Everyone should receive a minimum income to cover basic costs to allow for greater flexibility. The expanded child tax credit was another example: every US citizen received a child tax credit based on the number of children they had.[296]

This is where the universal approach can sometimes align with the justice perspective. If we are able to transform our society into one based on principles of justice, there should be *no barriers*—no wooden fence—to having a basic income, having a house to live in, receiving health care, being able to raise children in a safe environment, or receiving an education. So, while equity (and not equality) can be an organizing principle for our transformation work, we cannot overlook opportunities to work toward justice within our society. We have to consider and grow opportunities that allow us to guarantee access to basic human rights for everyone.

* * *

Through my work, I have gotten involved in several efforts focused on anti-racist organizational change. Anti-racism is a word that has gotten much attention since the 2020 uprisings, but it is an approach that has been long advocated for by activists, scholars, and others aiming to reduce racism in society. You likely have heard a famous quote attributed to Angela Davis: "In a racist society, it is not enough to be non-racist, we must be anti-racist." An anti-racist approach asks us to acknowledge that we live in a racist society. This book has provided ample evidence that opportunities, harms, and resources are very often patterned by race such that white Americans receive advantages and Black, Indigenous, and other people of color are disadvantaged. Racism in our past and present policies have created a vastly unequal society, with race as one of the primary determinants of opportunity and outcomes. In our news stories and politics, we also know that racist individual attitudes and actions are alive and well in this country. Given that is the reality, what would it mean if every single person in the United States could magically become not racist? Would outcomes magically become more equal? Would inequities melt away?

To answer that question, I love the powerful analogy that Beverly Tatum uses to describe anti-racism. She is the author of *Why Are All the Black Kids Sitting Together in the Cafeteria?* She writes:

> I sometimes visualize the ongoing cycle of racism as a moving walkway at the airport. Active racist behavior is equivalent to walking fast on the conveyor belt. . . . Passive racist behavior is equivalent to standing still on the walkway. No overt effort is being made, but the conveyor belt moves the bystanders along to the same destination as those who are actively walking. . . . unless they are walking actively in the opposite direction at a speed faster than the conveyor belt, unless they are actively anti racist, they will find themselves carried along with the others.[297]

If we could wave a magic wand and remove all racist thoughts and behaviors from people, the conveyor belt would keep moving. Racism would still exist in our society because it is baked into our history and how our neighborhoods, criminal justice, education, and financial systems operate. And that is why we need to take an explicitly anti-racist approach. Before we dive into what this means, we need to be explicit about what "racism" is.

Dr. Camara Jones is a leading scholar of racism and health and a hero of mine. Long before the COVID-19 pandemic brought greater awareness to racial health inequities, Dr. Jones launched a national campaign against racism from her platform as president of the American Public Health Association. To help us understand what exactly racism is, she offers this definition:

> Racism is a system of structuring opportunity and assigning value based on the social interpretation of how one looks (which is what we call "race"), that unfairly disadvantages some individuals and communities, unfairly advantages other individuals and communities, and saps the strength of the whole society through the waste of human resources.[298]

Let us take a closer look at that definition. First, she defines racism as a *system*, which, as she clarifies in her second sentence, is a critical perspective for understanding that our systems need to change rather than merely rooting out people we deem as racist in our society. Second, she says that it structures opportunity and assigns value based on race. This means that the opportunities that a person has access to and the value placed on their life or contributions is shaped by what race people perceive them to be. Third, these opportunities and values are unevenly distributed across the population, with some people experiencing disadvantages and others experiencing advantages. The specifics of who receives advantages and who receives disadvantages depends on the context. Generally, white people experience advantages while Black, Indigenous, and other people of color experience disadvantages. Light-skinned Black people may also experience advantages over dark-skinned Black people, and people racialized as Asian or Latino might experience advantages over Black people. It is critical to be clear about not just the harm that racism causes people but also the benefits and advantages it creates for people. Finally, the definition emphasizes that this system "saps the strength of the whole society."

While some groups—namely, white Americans—experience advantages from the system, it is also harming the broader society we live in. Millions of people are unable to reach their potential. They are unable to become a groundbreaking researcher, an inspiring teacher, a transformative community leader, a supportive neighbor, or an influential artist because the system held them back. It held them back by failing to provide an adequate education, by providing more funding for police than after-school programs, by exposing them to environmental toxins like lead, and by creating enormous barriers to health care. While the people of color being denied these opportunities are clearly harmed the most, even those of us who are white are harmed when people are not allowed to reach their full potential. As Heather McGhee's book *The Sum of Us* explains, our inadequate public infrastructure and lack of other public resources is the result of a system of racism that prioritizes denying Black, Indigenous, and other people of color access to these resources and opportunities, even if it means also denying white people those same resources.[6]

By highlighting that racism is a system, rather than a problem of an individual, Dr. Jones moves us away from focusing our attention on whether or not someone is racist. Instead, anchoring ourselves in this definition helps us to understand that everyone is affected (it "saps the strength of the whole society") and that to be anti-racist, we need to focus our energy on disrupting this system.[298]

If we use this definition of what racism *is*, then what does it mean to be anti-racist? Keeping Dr. Jones's definition in mind, to take anti-racist action means that we need to work toward *restructuring opportunities, reassigning value,* and *preventing the waste of human resources* using a racial equity lens that values and creates opportunities for racially marginalized communities.[299] She asks us all to (1) name racism, (2) ask "how is racism operating here?" and (3) organize and strategize to act.[298]

Anti-racism is a practice rather than a state of being. Remember Beverly Tatum's moving walkway?[297] We cannot ever just *be* anti-racist; we have to be taking action. Further, anti-racism is a praxis (remember that word from chapter 10?), which means it is a constant state of reflection and action.[300] This means that anti-racism is a lifelong commitment to critically reflecting on the choices we are making and actively choosing to take action to disrupt the system of racism. We are likely to fall short sometimes, but our ongoing reflection will allow us to identify how to move toward a sustained anti-racist practice.

If we focus our energy on trying to decide whether a person *is* racist or anti-racist, where does that leave us? It draws our attention to individuals rather than focusing on the systems. We do not want to absolve people with truly racist belief systems and actions, but it can be much more helpful to focus our energy on which choices or behaviors reinforce our system of racism and which choices or behaviors help to disrupt our system of racism. Or to use Tatum's analogy, which choices or behaviors actually help us walk fast enough against the moving walkway?[297] That helps us to keep the focus on the system and actions that move us toward a different and anti-racist society.

You might be wondering where other systems of oppression fit into an anti-racist framework. Addressing racism is good, but what about pervasive homophobia, xenophobia, sexism, transphobia, colonialism, ableism, and other systems that create advantages and disadvantages? Don't they matter? Absolutely. I understand this in two different ways, thanks to the insights from many anti-racist scholars and thinkers, especially those who have advanced the concept of intersectionality.

Intersectionality is a theoretical framework developed by Black feminist scholars and other women of color.[301-304] Their work helps us to understand that all these different systems of advantage and disadvantage work together and support one another. Colonialism created opportunities to build and enforce structural racism. Our system of racism, built over time, solidified the idea that there are people who are less worthy, and xenophobes and sexists build on that idea to oppress immigrants and women, respectively. But there are also Black women immigrants, and these systems of structural racism, xenophobia, and sexism intersect to shape their life in ways that are different from the experiences of other Black people, other immigrants, and other women. An intersectional perspective is fundamental to working toward anti-racism. A truly anti-racist approach would also help to undo these other systems of advantage and disadvantage.

Second, an anti-racism approach is not necessarily the best or only way to work toward equity and justice in our society. But it is an important way. Structural racism shapes much of the inequities and injustices that we see in US society and throughout the world. Therefore, directly tackling structural racism is a promising approach to working toward equity. Other systems of oppression also prevent people from accessing certain opportunities and also create hierarchy. It could be just as promising to engage a decolonizing or feminist or queering strategy (though, do not forget the point, made in the previous paragraph, about taking an intersectional approach). Tackling sexism or ableism without also considering the unique disadvantages that Black women or disabled Black people face could reinforce our system of racism (and vice versa). The important point is that you take steps forward toward a more equitable future using reflection and action to guide your steps forward to disrupt systems of inequity. There are many entry points, and an anti-racist perspective offers an opportunity to move to action.

Being grounded in these ideas of anti-racist practice—restructuring opportunities, reassigning value, and preventing the waste of human resources with a racial equity lens—can be an important guide for *how* we transform our society.

CHAPTER 13

What We Transform

Every moment is an organizing opportunity, every person
a potential activist, every minute a chance to change
the world.
—Dolores Huerta

Now that we have discussed *where* we transform and *how* we
transform, we are ready to talk about *what* we should focus our
energy on transforming. Remember the story of Katey Fahey
who spearheaded a constitutional amendment to Michigan's
state constitution to better enshrine voting rights and access to
voting for Michigan's residents. That is an example of making a
systemic change that will be long-lasting and have a broad impact. That is where we want to focus our attention when we are
thinking about what we transform.

Not every initiative is going to have the same impact that
Katey was able to have, but it is that mindset we want to focus
on. Remember the old adage: If you give a person a fish, you feed
them for one day; if you teach a person to fish, you feed them for
their lifetime. How can we bring that same long-term change
mindset into the transformation work we do?

We need to think more expansively than the simple fix. We
want to think about root causes. When Katey thought about

what needed to be transformed, she astutely recognized the importance of tackling a root cause. It is a lesson for all of us when thinking about what we need to transform to truly transform our society. This chapter describes several different areas we can focus on, including repairing and redressing past harms, improving democratic systems, shifting social norms, building community support systems, and disrupting power hierarchies.

* * *

We already talked about the long history in the United States of entrenching inequities, especially across racial lines. The US government and settlers took actions that resulted in a genocide against Native Americans. They also kidnapped Africans and placed them in perpetual bondage. Those sins were never fully redressed, and worse, the atrocities committed evolved into new forms of repression such as lynchings, redlining, forced removal from land, and numerous other harms. The legacy of those harms persists today, and before we can move on as a country, we need to consider how we can repair the harm that was caused.

In 1995, South Africa negotiated an end to its racist apartheid regime, and Nelson Mandela was leading a new African National Congress–led government. The new government was interested in healing the wounds of the past in order to move forward as a nation and enacted a law that would establish a Truth and Reconciliation Commission. Titled the Promotion of National Unity and Reconciliation Act, it could be a model for how the United States can move beyond the wounds of the past. The summary text of the legislation provides a roadmap for healing. It calls for the following actions:

(a) Establishing a complete picture of the human rights violations that occurred and sharing it widely with the country

(b) Granting amnesty to people who admit to and share relevant facts of the politically motivated harm they caused

(c) Giving victims an opportunity to share the violations they suffered

(d) Giving reparations and rehabilitation to victims

(e) Making recommendations to prevent future violations of human rights[305]

The bill also recommended a Committee on Human Rights Violations, a Committee on Amnesty, and a Committee on Reparation and Rehabilitation. In simpler terms, these committees would focus on what happened, forgiveness for perpetrators who confess, and repair for those harmed.

This type of commission was based on the ideas of restorative justice. When thinking about the vast harms committed during the apartheid period, Nelson Mandela and his new government could have focused on jailing all the people that caused harm. Instead, they adopted a restorative justice approach with the goal to focus on healing the wounds across society. While the process in South Africa was not perfect and received some critiques from different sectors, it represents an important strategy to address the harms of the past and move toward a different future.

There are differing views on whether South Africa's Truth and Reconciliation Commission was ultimately successful. Many believed it helped uncover the *truth* of what happened during the apartheid era, but some critics say that it fell short of providing the rehabilitation and reparations it promised. Other critics would have preferred retributive justice that punished perpetrators of abuses rather than the amnesty that was provided. But the commission helped the country move beyond its fractured past.[306] It offered the international community another tool for how a country can reckon with a harmful past and became a model for other countries. Canada subsequently established a Truth and Reconciliation Commission to heal from injustices perpetrated by the Canadian government against Indigenous people.

Thinking about the United States, we have yet to do any of the things that the commission aimed to do in South Africa. We do not have a full national record of the harms committed and agreement on what happened during our periods of chattel slavery and our history of genocide against Native Americans (or everything that happened afterward). Victims have not had the opportunity to share the harms they experienced. Perpetrators of harm have not been given the opportunity to confess and be forgiven. And we have not yet reckoned with repairing the harms.

We are likely a long way from taking these actions at a federal level. But there are innovative local efforts that could help build momentum for this type of action. The Kellogg Foundation has been leading work since 2016 to spread Truth, Racial Healing, and Transformation (THRT) into cities, states, and universities across the country. They backed away from the language of "reconciliation" because they correctly note that the United States never had a history where groups were in harmony with each other. Instead, it aims to *transform* those relationships. Kellogg describes THRT as follows:

> At its core, TRHT unearths the deeply held, and often unconscious, beliefs that undergird racism—the main one being the belief in a "hierarchy of human value." This belief fuels the perception of inferiority or superiority based on race, physical characteristics or place of origin, which then manifests in our systems, laws, policies and personal practices.[307]

The visionary and architect for THRT is Dr. Gail Christopher, a change agent and author of the book *Rx Racial Healing.* Dr. Christopher has built out this work across many locations in the United States, focusing on two core components: "narrative change (truth telling)" and "racial healing (trust and relationship building)." Narrative change refers to facilitating a more complete picture of our history and our present. It aims to change the way that our history and policies are depicted in our curricula, in the media, and in other major areas of our society. The overarching aim of this work is to be honest about the ways that a false notion of human hierarchy, based on race, has infected all realms of society. Racial healing refers to building relationships across racial lines; it recognizes the humanity of all individuals and dispels the myths of human hierarchy.

This work has gained some traction. In 2021, US Senator Cory Booker from New Jersey and Representative Barbara Lee from California introduced legislation to establish the first United States Commission for Truth, Racial Healing, and Transformation based on the framework advocated by Dr. Christopher.[308] This bill was proposed in the aftermath of the January 6, 2021, storming of the United States Capitol and intended to heal the divisions in US society. The proposed bill received numerous co-sponsors; unfortunately, as of the writing of this book, it ultimately died in committee.

Dr. Christopher talks about the importance of racial healing work this way:

> For America, we have to deal with what some people call our original sin—if that's what you believe—others call it our deepest wound and the soul of America. The deepest wound in America's soul is the fact that we became a nation because of this ability to devalue human beings. We built our economy, because of this ability to devalue human beings as a race of people. And we continue to let

that be the normative organizing theme of our society. And so we have to do that work."[309]

When we think about what we want to transform in our society, we need to be thinking about the healing, recognition, and repair work that Dr. Christopher refers to. We need to be thinking about the repair work, including financial repair for the financial harms caused to Black Americans and others. Since 1989, members of Congress have been working to persuade the US government to merely *study* the idea of reparations for Black Americans who are descendants of enslaved people.[310]

The late John Conyers, former US representative from Detroit, was the person who first spearheaded this initiative. Conyers was a civil rights leader and cofounded the Congressional Black Caucus. Like clockwork, Conyers would propose this bill to study reparations each new Congress. And each new congressional session, the bill would go nowhere.

Known as H.R. 40—because of the initial reparations concept of "40 acres and a mule," the false promise of reparations made to formerly enslaved people—the bill's text states this intent:

> To acknowledge the fundamental injustice, cruelty, brutality, and inhumanity of slavery in the United States and the 13 American colonies between 1619 and 1865 and to establish a commission to examine the institution of slavery, subsequently de jure and de facto racial and economic discrimination against African-Americans, and the impact of these forces on living African-Americans, to make recommendations to the Congress on appropriate remedies, and for other purposes.[310,311]

But the idea of repairing the harms of history proved to be too controversial for this bill to even make it out of committee for a vote during Representative Conyers's lifetime. In 2019 and 2021, the bill was put forth by Representative Sheila Jackson Lee and Senator Cory Booker. On April 14, 2021, the Judiciary Committee voted to move the bill to the full Congress, but it still failed to receive a full floor vote. Jackson and Booker tried again in 2023, but it failed.

Given the federal inaction on repairing past harms, some local governments are taking up the mantle. For example, the city government of Evanston, Illinois, passed a plan to give Black residents "reparations" for past discrimination and the effects of slavery. Each qualifying household would be eligible to be given $25,000 for home repairs or a down payment on a property.[312] Asheville, North Carolina, also allocated $2.1 million dollars to pay reparations.[313]

While this movement to acknowledge and address past harms is an important and necessary step, local initiatives are likely to be insufficient to truly repair the harms. Dr. William Darity is a professor at Duke University who has extensively studied reparations and highlights that effective reparations would need to close the wealth gap, which would require around $10 trillion to $12 trillion, well above what could possibly be paid by local governments.[314] Still, local efforts at reparations could soften the ground, allowing us to acknowledge past harms and genuinely engage in necessary repair work at a national level. It will be challenging to create a new society without first atoning for and repairing the harms, but our actions can help to pave the way for these efforts in the future.

*   *   *

Changing policies is important, but perhaps more important is thinking about how decisions are made and who gets to make them. We already talked about how gerrymandering can skew the results of an election at the legislative level by granting more power to a particular party than the breakdown of voters would indicate. Ending gerrymandering through nonpartisan citizen councils is a way to help change policy decisions. But there are many other ways we can transform our democratic systems to be more responsive to our communities.

One idea gaining some traction is the use of ranked-choice voting and multimember districts. In Portland, Oregon, in 2022, voters approved a ballot initiative that would transform city government into four districts, each with three representatives (instead of the typical one representative per district).[315] A form of ranked-choice voting known as single transferable vote will be used to select the three representatives for each district. Under the system, each voter would select their top candidate and then rank other candidates in order of preference. Any candidate earning 25% of votes would be elected as a representative. If a candidate earns more than 25%, their surplus votes will get shifted to the voters second choice to help determine who the three representatives are. The idea is that this style of voting and multimember districts can better represent the diversity within a district. Within the context of US partisan politics, a district that is 70% Democrat would typically have one representative that is a Democrat. But in multimember districts with ranked-choice voting, that district would likely end up with two Democrats and one Republican. It would help reduce polarization since the lower threshold for election creates space for a diversity of political views rather than just the typical two choices.

The proposed Fair Representation Act would implement the Portland system at the national level.[316] Under this proposed law, congressional districts would become multimember districts—largely eliminating gerrymandering—and ranked-choice voting would be used to select representatives. US Representative Donald Beyer has introduced this legislation several times in recent years, but it has gone nowhere. This type of legislation could benefit from the large-scale mobilization of voters who demand more equitable representation.

Beyond elections, there are other ways to think about resident participation in governance. What if residents had greater participation in budget allocations in their community? "Participatory budgeting" is one innovative idea defined as "a democratic process in which community members decide how to spend part of a public budget."[317]

One group in Central Falls, Rhode Island, put participatory budgeting into practice during the COVID-19 pandemic.[318] The federal government had allocated money for local governments through the American Rescue Plan Act (ARPA). The Central Falls School District used participatory budgeting to determine how the district should spend the ARPA funds coming its way. The district's superintendent or school board could have unilaterally made the budget decisions without any community input or perhaps hosted a community forum for ideas and then decided. But participatory budgeting takes it a step further and actually puts decision-making power into the hands of residents.

A group of 33 delegates, including 16 students and 17 parents, solicited ideas for how to spend the $100,000 of ARPA money in their district. They received numerous ideas, and then those ideas were voted on by a group of 146 members of the district community. The coalition Democracy Beyond Elections profiled this work and found that 97% of the delegates think participatory budgeting should continue in their district. Many delegates reported that it helped them feel more connected to their community, so it was successful in engaging residents in government processes. One parent delegate said: "In a way, my perspective has changed now that I was part of a process in which I knew what money was being invested into, knowledge that parents had no access to before. This makes me want more transparency about the funds and the way schools of [Central Falls] are run."[318]

Central Falls is not the only place experimenting with participatory budgeting. It has been implemented in over 7,000 locales around the world. In 2023, Seattle undertook one of the largest experiments with participatory budgeting when the city council allocated $27 million to investments in Black, Indigenous, and other communities of color, the result of activist demands made during the Black Lives Matter protests in the summer of 2020.[319] A working group of Seattle residents solicited ideas and developed them into feasible proposals. Residents voted on the proposals they most preferred. In the end, there were six projects that will be funded, including initiatives that support urban farming, a non-police crisis response program, and affordable housing.[320]

A group known as the Participatory Budgeting Project is helping to support the growth of this approach. One of its co-executive directors, Shari Davis, was profiled by the *New York Times* in 2022. Shari spoke about the potential importance and impact of participatory budgeting processes:

> How are budgets typically made? A guy or a group of guys makes some guesses based on last year's budget, and that's it—that's the budget. The money generally goes to big police budgets, or to a narrow view of what our schools need, or what education support looks like. Where it's not going is social services, or expanded opportunities for social work, or mutual aid spaces. It's not going into dedicated programming for Black, brown and trans youth. That's not a good or inclusive process. Community spending priorities don't get heard. People then get disillusioned, and eventually we see this narrative that they're apathetic. That's not it at all. It's that their engagement is inauthentic. Studies have found young people are more likely to vote in local and national elections after they were

involved in participatory budgeting, more likely to walk into a city-owned building, more likely to consider going into politics, more likely to speak to a public official, more likely to volunteer and more confident in their skills.[321]

Shari Davis and their colleagues are also thinking about how other democratic systems might change. They have been instrumental in the formation of Democracy Beyond Elections. This coalition is thinking deeply about how to engage in more participatory democracy where residents are involved at all levels of making policy, not just elections. They define it as "the policy-making process that invites community members to identify, develop, and decide directly on policy proposals."[322]

Outside the United States, there are numerous innovations that could be brought into the US democratic systems and way of governance. The think tank Demos Helsinki, based in Finland, imagines and works toward a "fair, sustainable, and joyful next era."[323] Its work is rooted in futurism, alternative ways of thinking about resident participation in governance, and sustainable policymaking for a transformative future. For example, Demos Helsinki conducts pilot projects on "anticipatory governance," a form of policymaking that tries to "balance between short-term needs and long-term vision: building resilience and driving transformation."[324] This model of anticipatory governance has been applied in North Macedonia in an effort to create migration policies that create needed protection, pathways, and solutions for refugees and asylum-seekers. Monica Sandri, a representative from the United Nations Refugee Agency in North Macedonia, shared her experience with anticipatory governance: "Change cannot be compartmentalized, so to be future-fit, we have to be open for a fundamental transformation to the way we work based on the commitment to look forward and be prepared while fostering participation, curiosity, courage, efficiency, and cooperative relationships."[325] Demos Helsinki is also creating new visions for participation in democratic systems with ideas like "humble government," which is a shift away from top-down decision-making, and by better integrating marginalized community members in ideation and decision-making.[326] Integrating these new ways of thinking about resident participation and governance are part of the transformation that we need to make a better world possible.

* * *

There is no policy in place that says that women in heterosexual relationships have to do more household chores than men, and yet women do 2.5 more hours of housework per week than men.[327] There is no policy that says we can't drop by a neighbor's house for an unplanned and uninvited hangout, and yet many Americans feel this would be inappropriate. And there is no policy that prohibits someone from wearing a shirt when it gets a big stain on it, and yet most people feel that a fully functional but stained shirt is no longer acceptable for public wear. These are all social norms in most parts of our society.

We have gotten a taste of the difference between norms and policy with the presidencies of Donald Trump. While he seems to have broken many policies while in office, many things that President Trump has done are violations of *norms*. Social media insults hurled by the president once shocked us because it was against our norms of how we thought a president should act. But it wasn't against the law, it was just against the norms of our presidency. When he did not release his taxes or medical records, he was shirking decades-long norms of presidential candidates. He was not breaking any laws. That is why in 2022, Congress tried to pass a law that would actually force presidential candidates to release their taxes so that voters could have a better sense of the financial entanglements a president might have.

While the consequences for Trump have been slippery, there are often real consequences for norms violations. There is a robust discussion and analysis of social norms within the social sciences.[328] For most of us, in deciding how to act, a person will consider the people in their social network whose opinion they value. Social science researchers call this your "reference group." Essentially, they are the people you are looking to for guidance in shaping your behaviors. Your reference group will vary depending on the context and type of action you are taking. Your parenting choices may be influenced by other school parents, but your decision about whether or not to participate in the office book club will be more influenced by your work colleagues.

Social norms can shape our frivolous actions that do not really matter. Social norms will partially inform our decision on how to greet someone: Will you shake hands, fist-bump, bow, hug, do that weird elbow grab thing, or use some other physical gesture? But social norms can be critically important for the changes we need to make as a society.

Perhaps this is easiest to see in the context of climate change. If we want to disrupt climate change, we certainly need policies to help drive us into a more sustainable economy. But we also need our societal norms to change. In the United States, our norms have created a consumeristic sprawl society that is accustomed to wasting resources and contributing to accelerating climate change. To work toward a more sustainable society, we need norms to start to shift, which can then drive demand for policy change and promote further change in social norms in a cyclical fashion.

In most social circles, it is *not* socially acceptable to be extremely wasteful of paper, to burn plastic bags, or to litter. These things are socially unacceptable because there is fairly widespread agreement that they harm our environment, and we

collectively want to avoid that. Yet it *is* socially acceptable to frequently travel by air, despite air travel being a major contributor to greenhouse gases. It is socially acceptable to buy and use
things like ziplock bags or plastic forks that you only use once
and then throw away (although, in many circles, this norm is
changing). It is socially acceptable to avoid mending clothes or
furniture and simply buy a new one and throw the slightly dam-
aged one in the trash. It is socially acceptable—and often socially
encouraged—to eat beef even though its production has an out-
sized impact on climate change compared to other foods.

These are all areas where social norms could shift to help us
make different choices. If your friends gave you side-eye when
you ordered a cheeseburger at the restaurant, you would be more
likely to choose the chicken sandwich or black bean burger. Importantly, a policy or tax discouraging eating cheeseburgers
might seem too paternalistic and restrictive, but changing norms
encourages that behavior in a more subtle way.

So how do we change norms? The good news is that we can
play an important role in our own social networks. Social norms
are built on three things.[328]

1. What do we think people who are important to us *are*
   doing?
2. What do we think people who are important to us *think*
   we should be doing?
3. How will I be rewarded or punished by those important
   people if I do (or don't do) something?

The key thing to remember is that *you* are likely one of those
people who are important to *someone else*. So, your friend's behaviors will be based on what they think *you are doing* and what
they think *you think they should do*. This means that to shape

norms, you might choose to be open with your friends about your own behaviors and your opinion about what you would like them to do.

The first one is easy. If you have purposefully taken action to reduce your carbon footprint (or disrupt racism or some other thing), tell your loved ones about it! Tell them why you think it is important and how you have been able to do it. This will make your loved ones more aware. Our loved ones often misperceive what we actually do. There are some famous studies about how most college kids think that their fellow students are getting drunk all the time, but the reality is much different.[329] Part of the reason is that the drunkard students usually talk about their drinking all the time while the nondrinkers seldom talk about their decision to not get drunk. So what college students hear are stories of people drinking all the time. Their mind makes the leap to think that everyone is doing that.

The same would likely be true about our choices to build a better world. Consider the example of air travel, a contributor to climate change. Let's say that you typically take one overseas trip a year, and you purposefully made the choice to swap one of those trips out every other year with a trip to somewhere that is just a two-hour drive away. You made this choice to reduce your family's carbon footprint. If you are not explicit about this choice with your loved ones, they will only hear how fun your trips are, and they are unlikely to conclude that you have intentionally reduced your air travel. Simply telling our friends some of the things we are doing to create a better world is a first step toward changing the norms in our social circle.

The second one is a little trickier because we likely are hesitant to express judgment on someone else. But oftentimes, when we express to important people in our lives not just what choice we have made but also *why* we made that choice, it makes it implicit that we think others should come to the same conclusion.

If we think it is important to avoid single-use plastics because of how damaging they are to the environment, it is reasonable for others to assume that this is not just an individual choice but something that we believe everyone should adopt.

Years ago, I visited my older sister's home outside Washington, D.C., and she changed how I think about table napkins. We joined her family for a casual dinner, and I noticed she had folded cloth napkins beside each plate. Until then, I mostly thought of cloth napkins as "fancy" items that you only found in nice restaurants or at dinner parties. As I was helping my sister clear the table and clean up the kitchen, I looked around and realized that there was no paper towel roll on the counter. I asked if she always uses cloth napkins, and she said, "Yeah, I just hate to always be throwing away napkins and paper towels, so we have this drawer full of cloth napkins and washcloths that we use." In hindsight, I am a bit embarrassed that I never really thought about that concept before. But every household I had ever lived in had a paper towel roll on the counter and set out paper napkins at mealtime.

My sister was someone important to me. I respected her and looked up to her. Knowing that she was choosing to use cloth napkins made me reassess my own choice to use paper towels and paper napkins. She never said out loud, "I think you should use cloth napkins at your house because it is more sustainable." She didn't have to. After that evening, I knew an important person in my life was eschewing paper towels/napkins for environmental reasons, and I assumed that she probably thought other people should, too.

The final piece of social norms is the anticipated consequences of not following in my own household what my sister was doing in hers. In this case, I did not think that she would socially exclude me, yell at me, or otherwise punish me. But, if I am honest, I did think that if I continued to use throwaway paper napkins, she and other environmentally minded people invited to my house would likely notice. We humans don't love it when people think we are wrong or making the wrong choice. Soon after that visit to my sister's house, we mostly stopped using paper towels and paper napkins in my household; we now use a set of cloth napkins. This was a relatively simple change, and it aligned with my values, so it was an easy change to make. The social norms nudge from my sister—and remember, she never said a word about it except when I asked—helped to speed along the process.

That subtle influence might not have worked as well for a bigger or more complicated change in my life. It would likely have required more than just one important person in my life sharing their behavior and expressing their opinion about the matter. But the point is that these small interactions with loved ones matter.

We can be micro-influencers in our own social networks. And if you have a platform to be a larger influencer because of your status, social media presence, or job title, you should seize it and share the choices you make that have a positive influence on the world. No need to be braggadocious or preachy—just be authentic and honest about some of the choices you are making to make the world a better place. Share with others that you called your representative to discuss an upcoming policy decision, you donated to a local organization, or you helped your workplace change a harmful practice. People who see you as an important person to follow will be subtly influenced by your actions.

Now, another scenario might arise in your life where you know you should be making a certain change but you have simply not been able to do it. For example, you might have read the research on how beef consumption contributes to climate change, and you would love to drastically reduce—or eliminate—beef from your diet, but you have yet to fully make this behavior change. You and your partner enjoy Friday date nights and going out for cheeseburgers at your local greasy spoon, and your summers are full of barbecues with friends where burgers are always on the menu. Plus, your mother-in-law makes a phenomenal meatloaf. You have cut back your consumption a little bit, but the opportunities to eat beef keep coming up. In this case, you have *not* made a specific change yet, so you are not necessarily in a position to share this choice with your loved ones. But you can still use social norms to your advantage.

Bring together your group of friends and try to change the norms within your group *together*. If you all stop eating cheeseburgers at the same time, then you know that you have social support for the decision. This may require a discussion with your partner about how to do this together. If you both genuinely want to reduce your beef consumption, then the temptation you feel to order a cheeseburger will be dampened by the disappointment you perceive your partner will feel. Collectively, choose a restaurant with a delicious and satisfying alternative on the menu. With your barbecue friends, you can share your goal and your reasoning (with evidence if needed). You can decide what change you are aiming for: Is it full vegetarian barbecues? Is it making turkey or black bean burgers available? Make the case and make the ask well before the actual event so that everyone has the time to mentally adjust and modify their shopping plans.

Examples for how social norms can help us spur people to action go well beyond environmental sustainability and climate change. What if after each mass shooting in the United States, the pervasive social norm was to protest in the streets, contact decision-makers, and donate to gun safety organizations? Sure, some people do this, but most Americans just shake their heads and remark on how sad and frustrating it all is. But in our social networks, we could communicate the expectation that we take action together. I have a friend who has planned family-friendly, postcard-writing events on behalf of reproductive rights or immigrant rights at a local playground. It is just as fun as regular gatherings, and we try to make our voices heard on an issue that is important to us. Once this becomes a norm within the social group, we can dedicate more time, energy, and support to do the work to make change on important policy issues.

As stated at the beginning of this section, norms are different from policies. This book has largely focused on public policies that are causing harm, not social norms. But social norms can be powerful on their own and are often pathways to policy change and a better world.

*　*　*

When it quickly became apparent that COVID would shut down the world as we knew it, many people lost their livelihoods. The privileged among us got to continue earning a salary while we worked from home. But too many people stopped earning a paycheck when everything shut down. It was at that point that people like Maria Militzer and other informal community leaders sprang into action and showed the power of mutual aid.

Maria grew up in Mexico and trained as a veterinarian, but her life took a turn when she moved to Michigan.[330] Maria initially worked cleaning houses and doing other odd jobs, then she became a Spanish translator at the hospital and eventually pursued a PhD in public health in her 40s. Maria had built a successful life in the United States, and she was dedicated to helping other Latino immigrants in her community to thrive.

While Maria was in graduate school, she began to organize her friends—many of whom were immigrants—to better connect them to social support and to fight for access to critical resources. She organized events to celebrate Latino K-12 students who were graduating. She helped parents register their kids for school and helped others file necessary immigration paperwork. She engaged in numerous other activities to help her community. Slowly, Maria and the other leaders she worked with developed this work into a nonprofit organization called Mexiquenses Unidos. When COVID struck, Maria and the other Mexiquenses Unidos leaders were ready to organize support for their community. They quickly mobilized to provide mutual aid. They showed up for their community.

Over the first few weeks and months of the pandemic, Maria and her group combined forces with other groups working with immigrants and Latinos in the area and attempted to plug all the holes that were created by the pandemic. People needed money, food, medical care, information, deliveries, transportation, social support, child care, and personal protective equipment. The government was stepping in with *some* resources but not enough. In April 2020, the government offered $1,200 in stimulus payments to all adults to help residents meet their needs during the pandemic lockdown. But some immigrants were ineligible for that support, and people like Maria creatively took action to fill the gap.[331]

The key was that the community members came together to help each other. Some could contribute money, some could contribute time, some could sew masks. Some could not contribute anything and just needed the help from their neighbors. But when the community came together to address needs, the community recognized the abundance that existed within.

When we think about the issues facing our society, the principles of mutual aid are key for overcoming them. Living in our siloed homes and either waiting for the government to provide resources or trying to bootstrap ourselves into accessing those resources just will not work. Too many in our population will be left behind in that model. We recognize that the people and institutions with resources generally will not provide for everyone equally. We need, then, to come together in mutual aid. To fill in the gaps, we need to share what we have with each other—especially with those who have less.

Dean Spade is one of the key thinkers (and doers) writing about mutual aid. He describes it this way:

> Mutual aid is a form of political participation in which people take responsibility for caring for one another and changing political conditions, not just through symbolic acts or putting pressure on their representatives in government but by actually building new social relations that are more survivable.[332]

Spade provides this key definition to help us understand the type of work that Maria was doing with her neighbors and an approach that we all can take to start building a better world. In Spade's writing, he also highlights a prime example of mutual aid by a social movement organization: the Black Panther Party.

In January 1969, leaders of the Black Panther Party did something that some people thought was both radical and threatening: they arranged free breakfast meals for children in Oakland, California. They solicited donations from local businesses and recruited volunteers to help prepare and serve breakfast for kids in their neighborhood. The Free Breakfast for Children program soon expanded to other chapters of the Black Panther Party across the nation. The program served as a cornerstone of the Black Panther's Survival Programs—including services like testing for sickle cell anemia, free ambulance, and legal aid—which intended to help Black communities meet their basic needs in the absence of government support and services.[333] Many experts agree that the successful Free Breakfast for Children program helped prompt the federal government to create a free breakfast program that is still in operation today.[334] It is an example of *mutual aid*, where communities build their own systems of collective care.

Like this example from the 1960s shows, mutual aid is not a new concept. It is one that has been practiced for centuries and millennia in different ways. But well-resourced people and communities have theoretically had less of a need for mutual aid. After all, institutions rarely exclude them from their resources, and they have enough money to purchase what they need. As a result, these communities have slowly shed some of the ties that bind people together.

During the pandemic, mutual aid proved to be the most effective way to get these resources to community members, especially people that are sometimes distrustful of formal government channels that can provide resources. Growing mutual aid—between neighbors, between colleagues, between parents—can start to transform our relationships to each other and ultimately build a different society.

A mutual aid approach urges us to ask: How can we build systems within our own communities to meet people's needs? Likely, there are already mutual aid activities going on in your community that you can contribute to. Mutualaidhub.org is one resource that tries to identify mutual aid networks across the United States. In my local area, there is a group that organizes a food pantry and a pull-over prevention program that helps immigrants and people of color with car repairs (like fixing a broken taillight) to avoid their being targeted by law enforcement.

It is also important to remember that mutual aid does not need to be large in scale to have an impact. It can be as simple as a few neighborhood families coming together to share after-school child care responsibilities or creating a neighborhood volunteer bank for neighbors who need assistance with a ride, picking up medications, or minor home maintenance. How can you *come together* with other community members in a spirit of sharing to work against the sense of isolation and individualism that is so pervasive in our society today? Mutual aid gives us a framework to start building toward a better world of collective care that will allow us all to thrive.

* * *

In so much of our policies and decisions, power is concentrated within a small group of wealthy individuals. Part of what we need to transform is how decisions are made and who holds the power. Ultimately, the *people* should hold the power collectively.

Paying attention to types of power can help us to change how we exercise power and build power together to make change. British social theorist Steven Lukes, building on the work of others, articulated the three faces of power.[335] They are summarized by Jonathan Heller and colleagues as follows:

1. Visible: *Exercising influence in the political or public arena and among formal decision-making bodies to achieve a particular outcome.*

2. Hidden: *Organizing the decision-making environment, including who can access decision-making and what issues are being considered by decision-making bodies.*

3. Invisible: *Shaping information, beliefs, and worldviews about social issues.*[336]

The three faces of power help us to understand that power is not just about who gets to make the decision (the visible first face) but also about how the decision is made (the hidden second face) and what information counts as relevant (the invisible third face). With this in mind, we can think about how we bring the power of the entire community to bear on all the faces of power. Communities should get to make the decision; they should decide how the decision is made and what information is relevant for issues that are going to affect them directly. For us to get to this place, we need to have tools to analyze power in our society.

Power mapping is one strategy that allows us to focus our limited resources effectively. It is helpful for identifying who the key players are for any given policy decision and determining where to focus tactics. Members of the University of Michigan's Detroit Urban Research Center taught me a version of power mapping that I have now incorporated into my own teaching and projects.[337] Let's walk through their approach to power mapping as an example of how to analyze power.

It is best to do a power-mapping activity as a group with other allies who are working toward the same goal. First, you begin by stating what the specific policy goal is. The more specific the better. For example, say you are trying to change a policy at the local high school. A clearly stated goal to "End the contract with the local police department to station police in schools" is better and more specific than "Keep police out of schools." Then, you want to do your research and find out who makes the decision on this particular issue. This is critical because the decision-maker or decision-making body will ultimately need to take action to change the policy. If you are uncertain about who the decision-maker is, then prioritize figuring it out before proceeding further. In this example, the district superintendent or school board would likely be the ultimate decision-maker on a contract between the school district and local police.

After you have specified what your target policy goal is and who the decision-maker is, you list all the groups or individuals who are connected to or affected by the policy. You might include the "district superintendent" and "school principal" as well as groups like the "Parent-Teacher Organization (PTO)," "student council," and "local police department." This is a brainstorming process, so there is no need to overthink it. Just put a group or person on your list if you think they might be relevant. Typically, each person or group will be written on a separate sticky note.

After listing all the individuals and groups of people that would potentially be affected by the policy, you start to think about where they fall on the spectrum from "opponent" to "supporter" and where they fall on the spectrum of "high influence" to "low influence" on the decision. For example, the school principal would likely be highly influential. You would want to rely on local knowledge and group relationships to help you understand whether the principal is a supporter or opponent or somewhere in between. If you are not sure, you can note that as something to further research. You go through all of your sticky notes and ask yourself:

- How much does this person/group oppose or support the policy?
- How much influence does this person/group have on the decision?

Then you place each sticky note on a board that looks like the one developed by the Detroit Urban Research Center, shown in figure 13.1.[337]

At the end of this power-mapping exercise, you have a board that gives you a visual representation of where different key players and groups are. This helps you to identify where the power resides. Yes, the ultimate decision-maker has a lot of power in the situation, but so do some of the other players that you have identified and can potentially leverage to help influence the decision-maker. In terms of actions, you can think about how you move folks along the support spectrum. For example, perhaps your local knowledge tells you that the teachers union falls in the middle of the oppose–support spectrum. They can see certain advantages of removing police from schools but also are

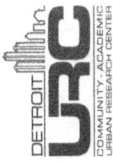

Power Map

Policy Goal: _____

Central Decision-maker: _____

Power & Influence

(High)

Major
Influence

Some
Influence

Can get
attention

Not on
Radar
Screen

(Low)

| SUPPORTERS | UNDECIDED/NEUTRAL | OPPONENTS |

Power & Influence

(High)

Major
Influence

Some
Influence

Can get
attention

Not on
Radar
Screen

(Low)

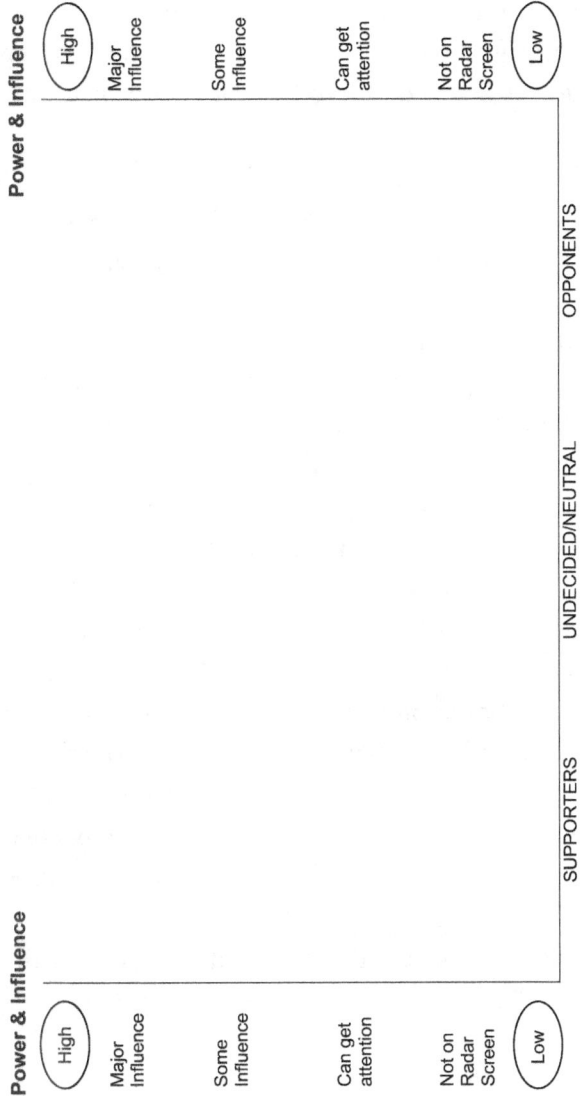

Definitions: Central Decision-maker: Has control over the decision
           Supporters: Are on our side, are for our policy change
           Opponents: Are against our policy change

detroiturc.org

Figure 13.1   Power map developed by the Detroit Urban Research Center. *Source:* Advocating for Policy Change Manual, Detroit Urban Research Center.

concerned about the increased burden teachers may experience if they do not have police to rely on for discipline. You also might identify that the teachers union is medium in terms of influence. They are not the decision-makers, and many demands made by teachers are ignored. But when teachers contact the superintendent, they are listened to, and they can easily bring attention to an issue.

Once you have things laid out, that is when the fun part happens, and you get to strategize your next moves. Obviously, the decision-maker is ultimately the person/group you want to influence. That person needs to agree with the change that your team supports. But how are you going to change their mind? (Or, if they already agree with you, what political dynamics are getting in the way of them acting on their position?)

This is when you can think about exercising the power you have built as a community to make the change that you want. This power is often based on a group of people organized to work collectively to achieve a certain outcome. If you determine that the school board is the decision-maker, then they are the ones that will need to vote to renew the contract with the local police department. Based on your research and local knowledge, you know that the school board is composed of seven members with equal voting weight. You know that the decision will be made by a simple majority vote. Thus, you need four votes out of the seven. You will now need to use your resources, relationships, and local knowledge to determine what school board members currently believe about the decision and who is most likely to be persuaded. This is where the rest of your power map comes into play.

You ultimately need school board members to vote to end the contract. You can approach this directly by setting up meetings with school board members, building relationships, sharing information that appeals to common goals, and making your case. This approach works best when there is an existing strong relationship with school board members. So, out of all the other key players whose names you wrote on sticky notes, who can you bring into the campaign to influence school board members? The superintendent is hired by the school board and head of the school district. This person is not a voting member, but their opinion is likely to be highly influential for voting board members. How can you either recruit them to be a champion for your position or, at the very least, make them neutral?

What are other ways to sway school board members? This is where you need to look again at who is listed on your sticky notes and your toolkit of tactics. Which sticky note might be influential on school board members? The PTO will be somewhat influential since school board members are reliant on votes to maintain their seat. What can you do with parents to help them rally around your cause?

If you know you need to find supporters among parents, you have many approaches you could use: write op-eds in local media, distribute information on social media, speak at PTO meetings, organize a protest or rally outside a school board meeting, meet one-on-one with parents, host a community forum, or many other options. Which one would best reach the PTO parents? As a group, you might decide that the best approach is to do a combination of tactics. You agree that you will meet one-on-one with a few of the PTO leadership members and try to build a relationship between your advocacy group and the PTO on this particular issue. You also agree to start posting information on the PTO Facebook page about the upcoming vote on the contract and some of the concerns that your group has about renewing the contract with police, sharing examples from other school districts that have successfully canceled their contract. These efforts will try to push members of the PTO more firmly into the "supporter" category.

Ultimately, by organizing in this way, you are building power for you and your community by bringing more and more supporters into your cause. You are disrupting the usual power dynamics where the power rests in the hands of a few. But by strategizing and exercising power, you can disrupt that status quo and help sway decisions. Ultimately, you can use this organizing and power to help change how decisions are made and what information is considered when decisions are made (e.g., do decision-makers listen to our most marginalized voices?). Transforming our society will require us to build collective power to transform where power resides so that policies better meet the needs of everyone and allow everyone to thrive.

*   *   *

The chapters in part III have covered key concepts and ideas for where we transform, how we transform, and what we transform. While not exhaustive, considering these different mindsets and approaches can help us to build the future we need.

CHAPTER 14

Conclusions

Making a Better World Possible

Oren Lyons is a member of the Onondaga and Seneca Nations of the Iroquois Confederacy and a member of the Indigenous Peoples of the Human Rights Commission of the United Nations. His powerful essay "An Iroquois Perspective," published in 1980, questioned the priorities of our society. He wrote:

> In one rationalization upon another, you continue the exploitation for wealth and power. But you must consider in the process and in choosing the direction of your life: How will this affect the seventh generation? The system that we have observed not only here but internationally demands exploitation; industrialization demands a power base. It demands work forces for the gods of profit. . . . What about that seventh generation? Where are you taking them? What will they have?[338]

I close this book with the questions that Lyons asks: What about that seventh generation? Where are you taking them? What will they have? Those are questions for us to collectively wrestle with and then chart a course of action. I hope the lessons from this book can guide us on the path to making a better world possible for our great-great-great-great-great grandchildren.

First, we need to be future-oriented. We need to ground ourselves in this seven generations perspective to prioritize an equitable future over the present-day emphasis on profits, materialism, and competition. This perspective shift helps to bring into sharper relief how unsustainable our current trajectory is and how transformation is needed to be able to hand a thriving society over to future generations.

Second, to work toward a thriving society, we need to imagine doing better. We need to shake loose from the constraints of the status quo and dream about a world where everyone's basic needs are met and people have equal access to opportunities. Cultivating our imagination for a better world is vital for the transformation that we need, and it requires shifting our perspective and being open to seeing things in new ways. The people who saw the Earth floating in space for the first time—a new perspective—helped to create Earth Day and new environmental protection policies. The new perspective shook them loose from the status quo and created a new sense of urgency. In the words of Mariame Kaba, we must ask, *What can we imagine for ourselves and the world?*

Third, we need to adopt a prevention mindset in order to recognize the policies that must be in place to get to that envisioned better future. A prevention mindset means we need to take these steps:

1. Identify the root causes of a problem (e.g., keep digging deeper).

2. Prioritize primary prevention (e.g., stop bad things from happening in the first place).

3. Focus on prevention that the affected group wants and needs (e.g., nothing about us without us).

These three tenets can help guide us to policies that will make a true impact and help everyone thrive. Recall the parable about the river. We cannot keep funding large-scale purchases of life-preservers; rather, we need to look upstream to identify the root of the problem and address it with our public policies. A prevention mindset makes good sense from an ethical perspective (we should minimize harms to people), an economic perspective (it is less costly if the harm does not occur in the first place), and a pragmatic perspective (preventing harms before they happen avoids headaches and heartache).

Fourth, we need to examine the different sectors of our society with this prevention lens to identify what types of transformations are needed. This book explored the specific sectors of health care, the environment, education, the criminal legal system, and public safety. I described how when we treat health care as a commodity rather than a human right, more people die and health care is ultimately more expensive. I shared how our education system can exacerbate inequities rather than minimize them. I presented research supporting the view that our lax approach to climate change and environmental regulations is harmful and shortsighted. I showed evidence that addressing issues of theft, violence, and drug use by putting people in jails is expensive, ineffective, and counterproductive. I detailed how public investments in policing could be better spent creating public safety through other mechanisms. And there are many other sectors, including financial services, agriculture, and the military, that warrant the same scrutiny, analysis, and expansive exploration of possible alternatives. When we shift our mindset and apply a prevention lens, we can better understand that we need these sectors and systems to fundamentally shift their approach in order to make a better world possible.

Finally, working toward a better world requires us to think deeply about where we transform, how we approach transformation, and what we transform. We need to first look within, at ourselves and our own communities and institutions, to identify how we can make an impact in our own backyard. We can be key change-makers within our communities by leveraging our cultural knowledge and relationships to organize for different policies and approaches. When we do this work, we need to adhere to certain guiding principles about how we approach transformation. These principles include knowing yourself and how you are connected to an issue, critical reflection, building relationships, working toward equity and justice, working in true partnership with others, maintaining an anti-racism approach, and adopting a long-term commitment to the work. These principles will help you stay the course toward a better future where all people can thrive. Finally, we need to be strategic about what we set our sights on transforming. We want to tackle things that can have a big impact, such as repairing historical harms, changing our democratic systems, shifting social norms, promoting mutual aid, and addressing power hierarchies. There are certainly other objectives to add to this list, but what I advocate is intended to be a guidepost on our journey toward a better future.

* * *

For me, I often think about the world that I will be handing over to my children and other people's children. I have a responsibility to the next generation for being a steward of this Earth and taking care of the house we all live in. I am inspired by the change-makers around me that have done the work within their own local communities to plant seeds for a better future.

A few years ago, I planted tulips in my front yard for the first time. The soil was rocky and clumpy, not exactly the fertile environment I was hoping for. But as the colorful leaves were falling from the trees, signaling the hibernation of living things that was to come, I had to trust that the tulip bulbs I was planting would survive through the winter and blossom in the spring.

I was uncertain and unsure that the seeds I was planting would change anything in the future. Looking at my soil, there was much reason for me to lack hope. And yet, I planted anyway and did what I could to help those planted bulbs grow into beautiful tulips.

When spring arrived, there was hardly any sign of life at first. But then, little by little, green tips poked through the ground and began to rise up. Not all of the bulbs I planted survived; some of them did not have the support they needed. But some of the seeds I planted in the past survived into the future, adding just a bit of beauty to the world that my children and others can enjoy for years into the future. A better world is possible, even if we are uncertain about the path we will take to get there. It just requires us to keep planting seeds today in service of a better world tomorrow.

Epilogue

2225

Ash's learning pod had been thinking about this day for years and specifically preparing for months. They were going to open a time capsule that had been placed in this building back in 2025 when people still called it a "school." Two hundred years later, though, it is so much more. During the 21st century, communities started to organize to make resources more accessible and oriented around community needs. It started with a few schools expanding the concept of the "school nurse" into health services for the whole family. But soon, with the isolation spurred by the 2020 pandemic and subsequent civil unrest in the decades that followed, some residents started to realize that their neighborhood schools could be a place where they start to build the new supportive community they all craved.

It started in just a few locations at first—some city neighborhoods but also hollowed-out rural communities that had been struggling for decades to find their way forward in the early 21st century. These innovators started to imagine and build their schools into hubs for connection, learning, and resources that would be available to community members from cradle to grave. Ash's learning pod exists within the Community Resource Collaborative. The building and the surrounding land houses several learning pods for young people, health services, a food pantry, a toolbank, a healing space, workshops for adults, vegetable gardens, and a nature space. You can visit the Community Resource Collaborative on any day of the week and you'll find an intergenerational mix of folks learning, working, and relaxing alongside each other.

Ash's learning pod included Ash and 10 other kids from their neighborhood, and they were all led by a mentor with assistance at different times from other neighborhood adults and older children. They had focused their learning over the past 3 months on the period 200 years ago when the time capsule was placed in the building. The novels they read for their lessons were those that were popular in that period. They studied artists and poets who were influential then, and they learned about the historical period of the Tumultuous 20s, digging into what the world was like when a pandemic collided with a fascist populist movement, a racial reckoning, and a rapidly warming planet.

Back at the co-op housing campus, Ash continued to churn over thoughts about what life was like back in the 2020s and attempted to discuss it with some neighbors. The learning pod mentor had explained that during that time period, people's understanding of their responsibility to each other and the planet was different. It was customary back then to compete with neighbors for who could have more things, even if that meant destroying nature or communities along the way.

The learning pod talked about how in some neighborhoods, people would compete for who had greener and plusher grass— dumping chemicals onto their yards and watering them every day—and each of these homes had their own gas-powered lawn mower rather than sharing a few community mowers in a toolbank. And those neighborhoods existed close to other neighborhoods that had no yard or green grass to worry about. Instead, they were worried about more pressing things like their hunger and safety.

There were so many things that sounded foreign to Ash. Grass was rare in their community today, reserved only for a few communal spaces where the whole community could relax or play games. Their homes and neighborhoods were full of self-sustaining native plants that did not need to be watered or mowed weekly. And how could people spend money on frivolous things like mowed grass when people nearby were struggling?

Ash struggled to comprehend the choices people made 200 years ago and felt like cruelty was pervasive during that time period. Ash asked, "How could they have treated each other like that? How could they have disregarded the gifts of planet Earth so carelessly?"

One of Ash's neighbors, Autumn, was in her late 50s and a history buff who collected objects from the 21st century. Autumn even came to their learning pod to share some of her artifacts and stories about the time period. Autumn described how people often left their homes in the morning, traveling great distances by themselves in vehicles that polluted the planet, then typically spent more than eight hours straight sitting at a desk with a computer. Then, they drove home—picking up some chemically processed and meat-heavy food on their way—and went to bed and did it all over again the next day. Autumn emphasized that they did this as part of their competition with neighbors to see who could have the most things and pass along the most resources to their own children. Autumn also shared that some groups of people would group together based on what they looked like or what country they belonged to and try to keep other groups of people from having more things.

What Ash struggled with the most was when Autumn talked about the people that were considered to be "winning" the competition against their neighbors. The winners had the biggest houses, the most stuff, and the most prestige. But they still went to work all the time and still wanted more things. That appetite to always want more, and to take from others to get it, was confusing to Ash.

Autumn also shared about the people in the 21st century that were losing the competition against their neighbors. If these people were sick, they usually had to avoid seeing a healer because they couldn't pay for it. Their basic needs were not provided by the community like they were now. They needed jobs, but many of those jobs did not pay them enough to pay for a place to live and food to eat. Some of them worked just as much as others, often 50 hours per week, but their employer paid them a wage that did not allow them to afford their basic needs. They were sometimes surveilled by government agents called "police" that had the power to lock people into a cage called a "jail." These agents even were allowed to shoot and kill people without any punishment (as long as the person they killed was poor or part of the group they used to call "Black"). Autumn explained that it was this way because the winners of the competition had a lot of collective power. They would group together and make rules that made it harder, or near impossible, for others to succeed.

Ash loved those evenings spent chatting with Autumn. In addition to being a history buff, Autumn was the lead cook for the communal suppers that helped ensure that everyone in their community had dinner on their table. Ash, like the other kids in the co-housing campus, had a role, and Ash's was to help the lead cook gather the materials and prepare them for cooking. In between moments of chopping and dicing, Autumn would check in with Ash about what they were learning in their learning pod. They had always had a good connection, but Ash became particularly enamored with the stories Autumn would tell about the early 2000s.

The real breakthrough for Ash came when Autumn explained some of the underlying values from the period. Values had shifted so drastically since then, mostly because the warming planet forced a crisis that could not be swept under the rug like so many crises before it. The deep-seated divisions in society slowly melted away as it became increasingly clear that broad collective action was the only way to save the planet from ecological collapse. That reckoning was what finally broke the stranglehold that capitalism had on society. Ash's ancestors 200 years ago began to question whether a system based on exploitation of both people and planet was a system that could carry humanity for another century. The capitalist system locked the people in the early 21st century into a mindset of more and more growth for more and more wealth creation for more and more stuff.

When Ash and her community gathered around to open the time capsule, they waited in anticipation of what might be in there. Ash thought about what they would put into a time capsule in 2225 for their descendants in 2425. Ash imagined putting in seeds, one of the quilts their community created to celebrate the winter solstice, poems written about their community, and a community-generated map of people, plants, animals, and resources. Ash thought those items might give their descendants a sense of their community life.

When their mentor led them in a ceremony to honor their ancestors and finally open the time capsule, Ash was surprised to see what was inside. While she understood what Autumn had taught her about the 21st Century values, the contents of the time capsule made it hit home. One by one, the mentor lifted out the item and announced it to the crowd that had gathered that day:

- *iPhone 16*
- *A hard drive with popular movies and television series*
- *Photos of city government representatives*
- *A newspaper detailing news of the day, including election disputes, wars, and a homelessness crisis*
- *Two outfits that were fashionable at the time*

There were a few more odds and ends that Ash did not understand. Ash soon became lost in thought. How could their ancestors be so different from them? Would Ash's descendants view them with the same confusion and critique that Ash viewed the people of the 21st century?

Overwhelmed by the past and reflecting on one's own responsibility to the future, Ash scurried away after the ceremony and slipped into the nearby forest trails to think more clearly.

Autumn had once told them that the forest had been clear-cut in the 19th century. What had once been a dense forest representing centuries of uninterrupted growth had been made naked and barren by a few humans who wanted to sell lumber to make a profit. But the community government in the 20th century passed a policy to protect some parts of the land from development and farming. New trees were planted and started to grow. Life continued to spring up, and roots became more deeply planted into the ground. The network of fungi connected the trees in a communication and collaboration network that enabled the trees and forest to thrive. Over the century, the forest returned to the thriving ecosystem it was before the 19th-century loggers came.

The beauty and sense of calm in the forest that Ash was experiencing right now was thanks to a prevention policy that stopped harm to this forest. But those same ancestors sometimes treated their fellow humans like a resource to be exploited. They did good, and they did bad. But some of those people planted seeds for today's world. Ash was connected to them. Ash's values and thinking today, in 2225, would not be possible without the ideas and action in 2025. There was an inescapable thread that connected Ash across centuries into the past and into the future.

Ash knew that 2225 was not a utopia. Ash and friends were pushing for their learning pod to better put into practice the concepts of kincentric ecology—the idea that humans are connected as kin to the living things around them—that was so prevalent in their lessons. There were still conflicts between families and communities that occasionally boiled over into a physical fight. But Ash's ancestors helped make a better world possible for them. How would Ash return the favor for their descendants in 2425?

* * *

To make a better world possible, we need to write the script for our future. Following on the wisdom of so many thinkers, sci-fi authors, and artists, we need to actively envision the future we want to see and the steps we must take to build it. Not in the abstract, but in full color and detail. We owe it to our great-great-great-great-great grandchildren who will live in the worlds we can only imagine.

Acknowledgments

It is wild how a book has just one name on the cover when there are so many who contributed to the ideas coalescing within its pages and helping to make it all the way to print.

Robin Coleman at John Hopkins University Press saw a book-worthy idea and a reluctant author and provided the encouragement and guidance to shepherd it all the way to completion. What started as an exchange on social media turned into a meeting, which turned into a years-long relationship to support writing this book. I'm grateful to you for helping me see the potential of bringing these ideas to a wider audience.

This book would never have existed without William Lopez. Observing him write his first book, *Separated*, showed me what writing is all about and introduced me to a version of public health academia that prioritizes writing for the general public. I'm indebted to the ways that William helped shape my thinking on some of the ideas presented in this book as well as my professional trajectory. His encouragement was crucial. I would not have pursued this endeavor without his input. He also gets credit as my writing therapist and coach, helping me navigate the tricky parts of writing and getting unstuck. He has always been a crucial thought partner for me, but I'm especially grateful for the way he has helped me navigate the book writing process.

A huge thank-you to Lindsey Thatcher, Hannah Mesa, and Wolfgang Bahr. Lindsey was a key sounding board for how to create a writing plan at a crucial stage in the process. Our regular check-ins during the initial drafting phase helped me get words on the page and move me toward a full draft. Hannah and Wolfgang provided research and reference management that allowed me to focus more time on writing.

Thank you to Jess Letaw, Rachael Zafer, Elyse Auerbach, and Ellen Parakkat, who were thought partners in developing my *Making a Better World Possible* newsletter. The newsletter is based on ideas in my book, but ideas sparked from creating the newsletter also found their way into the book. I appreciate each of you for pushing my thinking and helping me hone some of my ideas.

Melissa Creary and Whitney Peoples are my friends, colleagues, and co-conspirators in creating a better world. I have learned a tremendous amount from each of them about creating equitable and anti-racist systems and working toward change. Many of the ideas that we have discussed or worked on over the years are present here, and my own ideas about them have certainly been shaped by my connection to each of them.

I want to thank the community organizers and change-makers I've had the chance to work alongside, especially those within Public Health Awakened, the Coalition for Reenvisioning Our Safety, the Health and Power Organizing Project, and others. I learned about relationship-building, bold ideas like abolition, and strategizing for change. Being connected to and working with each of you has been like getting expert training in how to make a better world possible.

To the colleagues, community members, students, and friends I've worked with in public health, thank you for teaching me and guiding me along my path. This book reflects many lessons learned from our work together, and I'm lucky to work alongside each of you.

Acknowledgments

I am extremely grateful for the authors and creators who shaped my understanding of our world and history and public policies. A book like this brings together many different ideas, from many different people, and tries to stitch them into something new. I hope readers will use the references in this book to discover new books and authors that inspire them and expand their imagination and understanding of our world.

Thank you to my amazing supportive wife, Becca, who read some very early drafts and gave me the loving confidence to keep going. She also helped me find the time and space to fit book writing into our very full life. I draw inspiration from her commitment and compassion to serve others and create a better world. Thank you to my parents and sisters who have been my lifelong cheerleaders, each teaching me, in their own way, how to be compassionate, analytical, and action-oriented, all of which are themes that show up in this book. And to my children, Theo, Josie, and Greta, you were a wonderful distraction and respite from writing. Crucially, the goal of leaving you, your classmates, your cousins, and all other children with a better world motivated me to keep writing. I humbly hope that I am planting seeds that you and your generation will be able to harvest for a better future.

Appendix

Here are a few resources to help you dig in further to this history:

13th (documentary) by Ava DuVernay

1619 Project by Nikole Hannah-Jones

The Color of Law by Richard Rothstein

An Indigenous History of the United States by Roxanne Dunbar Ortiz

The New Jim Crow by Michelle Alexander

Racial Equity Institute (https://racialequityinstitute.org)

Stamped from the Beginning by Ibram X. Kendi

The Sum of Us by Heather McGhee

White Rage by Carol Anderson

When Affirmative Action Was White by Ira Katznelson

Seeing White (podcast) by Scene on Radio

References

1. Kelley, RDG. *Freedom Dreams: The Black Radical Imagination.* Beacon Press; 2002.

2. Vecsey C, Venables RW. *American Indian Environments: Ecological Issues in Native American History.* Syracuse University Press; 1980.

3. Seven Generations—the Role of Chief. Public Broadcasting Service. Accessed January 23, 2025. https://www.pbs.org/warrior/content /timeline/opendoor/roleOfChief.html

4. Origins & Trajectories. University of Michigan Inclusive History Project. Accessed October 24, 2024. https://inclusivehistory.umich .edu/our-research/frame/origins-trajectories/

5. Jones JB, Neelakantan U. *How Big Is the Inheritance Gap Between Black and White Families?* Federal Reserve Bank of Richmond; 2022. Accessed October 18, 2024. https://www.richmondfed.org /publications/research/economic_brief/2022/eb_22-49

6. McGhee HC. *The Sum of Us: What Racism Costs Everyone and How We Can Prosper Together.* Trade paperback ed. One World; 2022.

7. Vasquez Reyes M. The Disproportional Impact of COVID-19 on African Americans. *Health Hum Rights.* 2020;22(2):299–307.

8. Kaba M. *We Do This 'Til We Free Us: Abolitionist Organizing and Transforming Justice.* Haymarket Books; 2021:3.

9. Ackoff RL. *Differences That Make a Difference.* Triarchy Press; 2010:109.

10. Engler M, Engler P. André Gorz's Non-Reformist Reforms Show How We Can Transform the World Today. *Jacobin.* July 22, 2021. Accessed August 23, 2024. https://jacobin.com/2021/07/andre-gorz -non-reformist-reforms-revolution-political-theory

11. Rodriguez D. Reformism Isn't Liberation, It's Counterinsurgency. *Medium.* October 21, 2020. Accessed August 23, 2024. https://level .medium.com/reformism-isnt-liberation-it-s-counterinsurgency -7ea0a1ce11eb

12. Benjamin R. *Imagination: A Manifesto.* W. W. Norton; 2024: x.

13. Wallace, D. *This Is Water: Some Thoughts, Delivered on a Significant Occasion, about Living a Compassionate Life.* Little Brown; 2009:3–4.

14. Rogers K. Fifty Years After "Earthrise": The Famous Photograph Bolstered the Environmental Movement. *USA Today.* December 24, 2018. Accessed April 26, 2023. https://www.usatoday.com/story /opinion/2018/12/24/earthrise-50th-anniversary-photograph -earth-day-climate-change-column/2401196002/

15. Brown is quoted in Wise K. Anti-Racist Pedagogy in Art: A UNT Speaker Series Provides a Vision for the Future. *D Magazine.* February 4, 2021. Accessed April 26, 2023. https://www.dmagazine .com/frontburner/2021/02/anti-racist-pedagogy-in-art-a-unt -speaker-series-provides-a-vision-for-the-future/

16. Kelley RDG. *Freedom Dreams: The Black Radical Imagination.* Beacon Press; 2002.

17. Le Guin, UK. Speech in Acceptance of the National Book Foundation Medal for Distinguished Contribution to American Letters. November 19, 2014. Accessed October 18, 2024. https://www .ursulakleguin.com/nbf-medal

18. Arikha N. *Passions and Tempers: A History of the Humours.* Harper Perennial; 2008.

19. Morens DM. Death of a President. *N Engl J Med.* 1999;341(24):1845– 1850. https://www.doi.org/10.1056/NEJM199912093412413

20. Michigan Civil Rights Commission. *The Flint Water Crisis: Systemic Racism Through the Lens of Flint: Report of the Michigan Civil Rights Commission, February 17, 2017.* Michigan Department of Civil Rights. 2017. Accessed February 22, 2025. https://www.michigan .gov/-/media/Project/Websites/mdcr/mcrc/reports/2017/flint-crisis -report-edited.pdf?rev=4601519b3af345cfb9d468ae6ece9141

21. Incarceration Trends in Michigan. Vera Institute of Justice; 2019. https://www.vera.org/downloads/pdfdownloads/state-incarceration -trends-michigan.pdf

22. Historic Flint Water Civil Settlement Approved by Genesee County Circuit Court. Michigan Department of Attorney General. March 21, 2023. https://www.michigan.gov/ag/news/press-releases/2023/03/21/historic-flint-water-civil-settlement-approved-by-genesee-county-circuit-court

23. Copeny M (@LittleMissFlint). I'm 11. My generation will fix this mess of a government. Watch us. Posted on X. October 6, 2018. https://twitter.com/littlemissflint/status/1048677585704701953

24. Meyer K. Asked and Answered: President Obama Responds to an Eight-Year-Old Girl from Flint. Obama White House Archives. April 27, 2016. Accessed April 26, 2023. https://obamawhitehouse.archives.gov/blog/2016/04/27/asked-and-answered-president-obama-responds-eight-year-old-girl-flint

25. Associated Press. Fact Check: Obama, Trump Both Had Role in Flint Water Relief. *Michigan Radio*. March 27, 2017. Accessed April 26, 2023. https://www.michiganradio.org/politics-government/2017-03-27/fact-check-obama-trump-both-had-role-in-flint-water-relief

26. Fleming PJ, Spolum MM, Lopez WD, Galea S. The Public Health Funding Paradox: How Funding the Problem and Solution Impedes Public Health Progress. *Public Health Rep.* 2020;136(1):10–13. https://www.doi.org/10.1177/0033354920969172

27. U.S. Department of Health and Human Services. Fiscal Year 2024: Budget in Brief., D.C., 2023. Accessed February 22, 2025. https://www.hhs.gov/about/budget/fy2024/index.html

28. Dawes DE, Williams DR. *The Political Determinants of Health.* Johns Hopkins University Press; 2020.

29. McGhee H. *The Sum of Us: What Racism Costs Everyone and How We Can Prosper Together.* One World; 2022.

30. New York Times (@nytimes). Researchers who study Type 2 diabetes have reached a stark conclusion. Posted on X. October 5, 2022. Accessed April 27, 2023. https://twitter.com/nytimes/status/1577740437145649154?s=20&t=aazB3cioPPmmFZ2QcEP0Xg. The original New York Times article is by Roni Caryn Rabin and is titled "Medical Care Alone Won't Halt the Spread of Diabetes, Scientists Say." It can be found at https://www.nytimes.com/2022/10/05/health/diabetes-prevention-diet.html?smtyp=cur&smid=tw-nytimes https://www.nytimes.com/2022/10/05/health/diabetes-prevention-diet.html.

31. National Research Council, Institute of Medicine, Woolf SH, Aron L. Public Health and Medical Care Systems. In *U.S. Health in International Perspective: Shorter Lives, Poorer Health*. National Academies Press; 2013. Accessed December 4, 2023. https://www.ncbi.nlm.nih.gov/books/NBK154484/

32. Ewing R, Schmid T, Killingsworth R, Zlot A, Raudenbush S. Relationship Between Urban Sprawl and Physical Activity, Obesity, and Morbidity. *Am J Health Promot*. 2003;18(1):47–57. https://doi.org/10.4278/0890-1171-18.1.47

33. Murray S. Poverty and Health. *CMAJ*. 2006;174(7):923. https://doi.org/10.1503/cmaj.060235

34. Link BG, Phelan JC. Social Conditions as Fundamental Causes of Disease. *Journal of Health and Social Behavior*. 1995;35(Extra Issue):80–94.

35. Davis AY. *Women, Culture & Politics*. Knopf Doubleday Publishing Group; 2011.

36. Fresques H. Doctors Prescribe More of a Drug If They Receive Money from a Pharma Company Tied to It. *ProPublica*. December 20, 2019. Accessed May 21, 2023. https://www.propublica.org/article/doctors-prescribe-more-of-a-drug-if-they-receive-money-from-a-pharma-company-tied-to-it

37. Himmelstein DU, Lawless RM, Thorne D, Foohey P, Woolhandler S. Medical Bankruptcy: Still Common Despite the Affordable Care Act. *Am J Public Health*. 2019;109(3):431–433. https://www.doi.org/10.2105/AJPH.2018.304901

38. Fact Sheet No. 31: The Right to Health. United Nations Office of the High Commissioner for Human Rights (OHCHR). June 1, 2008. Accessed December 4, 2023. https://www.ohchr.org/en/publications/fact-sheets/fact-sheet-no-31-right-health

39. Americans Have No Right to Healthcare. January 31, 2022. Accessed December 5, 2023. https://www.medpagetoday.com/opinion/second-opinions/96938

40. Bonis PA. Health Care's Shift from Covenant to Commodity Comes with Consequences. STAT. September 9, 2022. Accessed December 5, 2023. https://www.statnews.com/2022/09/09/health-cares-shift-from-covenant-to-commodity-comes-with-consequences/

References

41. 1947 Pre-WHO Years. World Health Organization. Accessed January 18, 2025. https://apps.who.int/iris/bitstream/handle/10665/126402/1947.pdf

42. World Health Organization. *Constitution of the World Health Organization.* 1948. Accessed January 18, 2025. http://apps.who.int/gb/bd/PDF/bd47/EN/constitution-en.pdf

43. "My Most Important Task" Eleanor Roosevelt and the Universal Declaration of Human Rights. Roosevelt House Public Policy Institute at Hunter College. Accessed December 13, 2023. https://www.roosevelthouse.hunter.cuny.edu/exhibits/my-most-important-task/

44. Black A. Compelled to Act: Eleanor Roosevelt, a Fearful World and an International Vision of Human Rights. United Nations. December 8, 2023. Accessed December 13, 2023. https://www.un.org/en/un-chronicle/compelled-act-eleanor-roosevelt-fearful-world-and-international-vision-human-rights

45. United Nations. Universal Declaration of Human Rights. Accessed December 5, 2023. https://www.un.org/en/about-us/universal-declaration-of-human-rights

46. Gruskin S, Mills EJ, Tarantola D. History, Principles, and Practice of Health and Human Rights. *Lancet.* 2007;370(9585). https://www.doi.org/10.1016/S0140-6736(07)61200-8

47. Christopher AS, Caruso D. Promoting Health as a Human Right in the Post-ACA United States. *AMA J Ethics.* 2015;17(10):958–965. https://www.doi.org/10.1001/journalofethics.2015.17.10.msoc1-1510

48. Tolbert J, Cervantes S, Bell C, and Damico A. *Key Facts about the Uninsured Population.* KFF; San Francisco, 2024. Accessed February 23, 2025. https://www.kff.org/uninsured/issue-brief/key-facts-about-the-uninsured-population/

49. Status of State Medicaid Expansion Decisions. KFF; San Francisco, 2025. Accessed February 23, 2025. https://www.kff.org/status-of-state-medicaid-expansion-decisions/

50. Broaddus M, Aron-Dine A. Medicaid Expansion Has Saved at Least 19,000 Lives, New Research Finds. Center on Budget and Policy Priorities. November 6, 2019. Accessed December 5, 2023. https://www.cbpp.org/research/health/medicaid-expansion-has-saved-at-least-19000-lives-new-research-finds

51. Sharara N, Adam V, Crott R, Barkun AN. The Costs of Colonoscopy in a Canadian Hospital Using a Microcosting Approach. *Can J Gastroenterol.* 2008;22:565–570. https://www.doi.org/10.1155/2008/854984

52. Survey of Household Economics and Decisionmaking. Board of Governors of the Federal Reserve System. Accessed December 5, 2023. https://www.federalreserve.gov/consumerscommunities/shed.htm

53. Kenworthy N, Igra M. Medical Crowdfunding and Disparities in Health Care Access in the United States, 2016–2020. *Am J Public Health.* 2022;112(3):491–498. https://www.doi.org/10.2105/AJPH .2021.306617

54. Tolbert J, Drake P, Damico A. Key Facts About the Uninsured Population. KFF. December 19, 2022. Accessed December 13, 2023. https://www.kff.org/uninsured/issue-brief/key-facts-about-the -uninsured-population/

55. Bennett N, Eggleston J, Mykyta L, Sullivan B. Who Had Medical Debt in the United States? United States Census Bureau. Accessed December 13, 2023. https://www.census.gov/library/stories/2021 /04/who-had-medical-debt-in-united-states.html

56. Tikkanen R, Abrams MK. U.S. Health Care from a Global Perspective, 2019: Higher Spending, Worse Outcomes? The Commonwealth Fund. January 30, 2020. https://www.doi.org/10.26099/7avy-fc29

57. Waldrop T. The Truth on Wait Times in Universal Coverage Systems. Center for American Progress. October 18, 2019. Accessed May 21, 2023. https://www.americanprogress.org/article/truth-wait-times -universal-coverage-systems/

58. Marks C. Inside the American Medical Association's Fight over Single-Payer Health Care. *The New Yorker.* February 22, 2022. Accessed December 6, 2023. https://www.newyorker.com/science /annals-of-medicine/the-fight-within-the-american-medical -association

59. Current Health Expenditure per Capita (Current US$): Costa Rica, United States. World Bank Open Data. April 7, 2023. Accessed May 21, 2023. https://data.worldbank.org

60. Gawande A. Costa Ricans Live Longer Than We Do. What's the Secret? *The New Yorker.* August 23, 2021. Accessed May 21, 2023. https://www.newyorker.com/magazine/2021/08/30/costa-ricans -live-longer-than-we-do-whats-the-secret

61. National Center for Health Statistics. Table HExpType. National Health Expenditures, Average Annual Percent Change, and Percent Distribution, by Type of Expenditure: United States, Selected Years 1960–2019. 2021–2020. https://www.cdc.gov/nchs/data/hus/2020 -2021/HExpType.pdf

62. Whitman S, Good G, Donoghue ER, Benbow N, Shou W, Mou S. Mortality in Chicago Attributed to the July 1995 Heat Wave. *Am J Public Health*. 1997;87(9):1515–1518.

63. Kunkel KE, Changnon SA, Reinke BC, Arritt RW. The July 1995 Heat Wave in the Midwest: A Climatic Perspective and Critical Weather Factors. *Bulletin of the American Meteorological Society*. 1996; Jul;77(7):1507–1518.

64. Klinenberg E. *Heat Wave: A Social Autopsy of Disaster in Chicago*. University of Chicago press; 2015.

65. Independent Lens. *Cooked: Survival by Zip Code*. PBS; 2020. Accessed December 13, 2023. https://www.pbs.org/independentlens /documentaries/cooked-survival-by-zip-code/

66. Cusick D, E&E News. Chicago Learned Climate Lessons from Its Deadly 1995 Heat Wave. *Scientific American*. July 16, 2020. Accessed December 8, 2023. https://www.scientificamerican.com/article /chicago-learned-climate-lessons-from-its-deadly-1995-heat-wave1/

67. Kaplan S, Ba Tran A. Nearly 1 in 3 Americans Experienced a Weather Disaster This Summer. *Washington Post*. September 4, 2021. Accessed December 8, 2023. https://www.washingtonpost.com/climate-environ ment/2021/09/04/climate-disaster-hurricane-ida/

68. Chicago—Lowest Temperature for Each Year. *Current Results*. Accessed December 8, 2023. https://www.currentresults.com /Yearly-Weather/USA/IL/Chicago/extreme-annual-chicago-low -temperature.php

69. *February 2021 Winter Storm-Related Deaths—Texas*. Texas Department of State Health Services; December 2021. https://www.dshs .texas.gov/sites/default/files/news/updates/SMOC_FebWinterStorm _MortalitySurvReport_12-30-21.pdf

70. Golding G, Kumar A, Mertens K. Cost of Texas' 2021 Deep Freeze Justifies Weatherization. Federal Reserve Bank of Dallas. April 15, 2021. Accessed December 8, 2023. https://www.dallasfed.org /research/economics/2021/0415

71. Douglas E. Winters Get Warmer with Climate Change. So What Explains Texas' Cold Snap in 2021? *Texas Tribune.* December 14, 2021. Accessed December 8, 2023. https://www.texastribune.org /2021/12/14/winter-weather-texas-climate-change/

72. Cohen J, Agel L, Barlow M, Garfinkel CI, White I. Linking Arctic Variability and Change with Extreme Winter Weather in the United States. *Science.* 2021;373(6559):1116–1121. https://www.doi.org /10.1126/science.abi9167

73. Hayhoe K, Wuebbles D. *Climate Change and Chicago: Projections and Potential Impacts.* City of Chicago. Accessed May 6, 2025. https://www.chicago.gov/content/dam/city/progs/env/CCAP/ Chicago_climate_impacts_report_Executive_Summary.pdf

74. Dee SG. Scientists Understood Physics of Climate Change in the 1800s—Thanks to a Woman Named Eunice Foote. *The Conversation.* July 22, 2021. Accessed March 20, 2023. http://theconversation.com /scientists-understood-physics-of-climate-change-in-the-1800s -thanks-to-a-woman-named-eunice-foote-164687

75. Foote E. Circumstances Affecting the Heat of the Sun's Rays. *American Journal of Science and Arts.* 1856;22:382–383.

76. Lindsey R. Climate Change: Atmospheric Carbon Dioxide. *NOAA Climate.gov.* May 12, 2023. Accessed December 11, 2023. http:// www.climate.gov/news-features/understanding-climate/climate -change-atmospheric-carbon-dioxide

77. Arrhenius S. On the Influence of Carbonic Acid in the Air upon the Temperature of the Ground. *The London, Edinburgh, and Dublin Philosophical Magazine and Journal of Science.* 1896;Apr 1; 41(251):237–276.

78. Molena F. Remarkable Weather of 1911. *Popular Mechanics.* March 1912:339–342. The quote goes on to say that "since burning coal produces carbon dioxide it may be inquired whether the enormous use of the fuel in modern times may not be an important factor in filling the atmosphere with this sub-stance, and consequently indirectly raising the temperature of the earth."

79. Ritchie H, Roser M. CO_2 Emissions. Published online at OurWorld-inData.org. 2020. Accessed February 24, 2025. https://ourworldin data.org/co2-emissions

80. Franta B. What Big Oil Knew About Climate Change, in Its Own Words. *The Conversation*. October 28, 2021. Accessed December 8, 2023. http://theconversation.com/what-big-oil-knew-about-climate-change-in-its-own-words-170642.

81. President's Science Advisory Committee. *Restoring the Quality of Our Environment*. The White House; 1965. Accessed December 8, 2023. https://www.climatefiles.com/climate-change-evidence/presidents-report-atmospher-carbon-dioxide/

82. *Electric Vehicles and Other Alternatives to the Internal Combustion Engine: Hearings Before the United States Senate Committee on Commerce, Subcommittee on Air and Water Pollution, and Senate Committee on Public Works, Ninetieth Congress, First Session, on Mar. 14–17, Apr. 10, 1967*. US Government Printing Office; 1967.

83. Millan L. Climate Change Linked to 5 Million Deaths a Year, New Study Shows. *Bloomberg*. July 7, 2021. Accessed December 8, 2023. https://www.bloomberg.com/news/articles/2021-07-07/climate-change-linked-to-5-million-deaths-a-year-new-study-shows

84. Daly M, Borenstein, S. Trump Signs Executive Order Directing US Withdrawal from the Paris Climate Agreement—Again. Associated Press. Accessed February 25, 2025. https://apnews.com/article/trump-paris-agreement-climate-change-788907bb89fe307a964be757313cdfb0

85. Cumulative Carbon Dioxide Emissions from Fossil Fuel Combustion Worldwide from 1750 to 2021, by Major Country. *Statista*. Accessed December 8, 2023. https://www.statista.com/statistics/1007454/cumulative-co2-emissions-worldwide-by-country/

86. Rahman MM, Alam K, Velayutham E. Is Industrial Pollution Detrimental to Public Health? Evidence from the World's Most Industrialised Countries. *BMC Public Health*. 2021;21(1):1175. https://www.doi.org/10.1186/s12889-021-11217-6

87. Stanton R. Charles Gelman, Founder of Gelman Sciences, Dies at 86. *MLive.com*. April 17, 2018. Accessed December 8, 2023. https://www.mlive.com/news/ann-arbor/2018/04/charles_gelman_founder_of_gelm.html

88. Monson, L. History of the Pall-Gelman Dioxane Groundwater Contamination Cleanup. Ann Arbor District Library. Accessed February 25, 2025. https://aadl.org/features/pall_gelman_cleanup

89. Dioxane Discovered from Gelman Sciences. The Ecology Center. Accessed December 8, 2023. https://ecologycenter.umhistorylabs.lsa .umich.edu/s/ecohistory/page/dioxane-discovered-from-gelman -sciences

90. Leif Bates K. Pollution Suit Thrown Out; Gelman Wins. *Ann Arbor News*. July 26, 1991. Accessed December 8, 2023. https://aadl.org/aa _news_19910726_pa1_back_page-pollution_suit_thrown_out _gelman_wins

91. Smolcic Larson L. EPA Says Ann Arbor-Area Dioxane Plume Eligible to Become Superfund Site. *MLive.com*. November 3, 2023. Accessed December 9, 2023. https://www.mlive.com/news/ann -arbor/2023/11/epa-says-ann-arbor-area-dioxane-plume-eligible-to -become-superfund-site.html

92. Bullard RD. The Threat of Environmental Racism. *Natural Resources & Environment*. 1993;7(3):23–56.

93. Census Profile: 48217. *Census Reporter*. Accessed December 9, 2023. http://censusreporter.org/profiles/86000US48217-48217/

94. Landrum T. I Live in One of America's Most Polluted Zip Codes. *Medium*. July 8, 2020. Accessed December 9, 2023. https:// evergreenaction.medium.com/i-live-in-one-of-americas-most -polluted-zip-codes-beb12a6bcde

95. Lerner S. *Sacrifice Zones: The Front Lines of Toxic Chemical Exposure in the United States*. MIT Press; 2012.

96. Shaw A, Younes L. The Most Detailed Map of Cancer-Causing Industrial Air Pollution in the U.S. *ProPublica*. November 2, 2021. Accessed December 9, 2023. https://projects.propublica.org /toxmap/

97. Hopkins H. Racism Is Killing the Planet. *Sierra*. June 8, 2020. Accessed December 9, 2023. https://www.sierraclub.org/sierra /racism-killing-planet

98. Peterson M. The Sad Irony of "Not In My Backyard" (NIMBY). American Institute for Economic Research. January 2, 2024. Accessed October 18, 2024. https://aier.org/article/the-sad-irony -of-not-in-my-backyard-nimby/

99. Permit Denied: Southeast Side Community Organizers Win Environmental Justice Fight. Health & Medicine Policy Research Group. February 25, 2022. Accessed December 9, 2023.

https://hmprg.org/news/permit-denied-southeast-side-community
-organizers-win-environmental-justice-fight/

100. Robinson KS. *Ministry for the Future.* 1st paperback ed. Orbit; 2021.

101. Summary: S.Res.173—A Resolution Recognizing the Duty of the
Federal Government to Create a Green New Deal. *Congressional
Research Service.* April 25, 2023. Accessed December 9, 2023.
https://www.congress.gov/bill/118th-congress/senate-resolution/173.

102. Atkin E. The Democrats Stole the Green Party's Best Idea. *The New
Republic.* February 22, 2019. Accessed December 9, 2023. https://
newrepublic.com/article/153127/democrats-stole-green-partys-best
-idea

103. The Red Nation (Albuquerque, New Mexico), ed. *The Red Deal:
Indigenous Action to Save Our Earth.* Common Notions; 2021.

104. Kimmerer RW. *Braiding Sweetgrass: Indigenous Wisdom, Scientific Knowledge, and the Teachings of Plants.* Milkweed Editions;
2020.

105. Salmón E. Kincentric Ecology: Indigenous Perceptions of the
Human-Nature Relationship. *Ecological Applications.* 2000;10(5):
1327–1332. https://www.doi.org/10.2307/2641288

106. Estimating Costs. Financial Aid University of Michigan. Accessed
December 11, 2023. https://finaid.umich.edu/getting-started
/estimating-costs

107. Stevens ML, Armstrong EA, Arum R. Sieve, Incubator, Temple,
Hub: Empirical and Theoretical Advances in the Sociology of Higher
Education. *Annu Rev Sociol.* 2008;34(1):127–151. https://www.doi
.org/10.1146/annurev.soc.34.040507.134737

108. Picker L. The Effects of Education on Health. National Bureau of
Economic Research. March 2007. Accessed March 20, 2023.
https://www.nber.org/digest/mar07/effects-education-health

109. Hanson M. US Public Education Spending Statistics. *Educationdata
.org.* September 8, 2023. Accessed December 8, 2023. https://
educationdata.org/public-education-spending-statistics

110. Hanson M. Average Cost of College over Time: Yearly Tuition
Since 1970. *Educationdata.org.* January 9, 2022. Accessed
December 8, 2023. https://educationdata.org/average-cost-of
-college-by-year

111. Hanson, M. Average Cost of College by Country. EducationData.org. January 21, 2025. Accessed May 2, 2025. https://educationdata.org/average-cost-of-college-by-country.

112. Student Funding Larger Share of Higher Education After Recessions. Center on Budget and Policy Priorities. Accessed December 8, 2023. https://www.cbpp.org/student-funding-larger-share-of-higher-education-after-recessions

113. White GB. The Mental and Physical Toll of Student Loans. *The Atlantic*. February 2, 2015. Accessed December 8, 2023. https://www.theatlantic.com/business/archive/2015/02/the-mental-and-physical-toll-of-student-loans/385032/

114. Who Is Most Affected by the School to Prison Pipeline? American University. February 24, 2021. Accessed February 25, 2025. https://soeonline.american.edu/blog/school-to-prison-pipeline/

115. Erwin B, Keily T, Peisach, L. *State Policies to Advance Student-Centered Pathways. Policy Brief*. Education Commission of the States; 2024.

116. Weller C. Eight Reasons Finland's Education System Puts the US Model to Shame. *The Independent*. January 8, 2018. Accessed December 8, 2023. https://www.independent.co.uk/news/education/education-news/finland-education-system-schools-model-superior-us-helsinki-children-a8147426.html

117. Sanders B, Jayapal P. *College for All Act of 2023*. S. 1963/H.R. 4117, 118th Cong, 1st Sess (2023–2024).

118. State-Funded Pre-Kindergarten: What the Evidence Shows. Assistant Secretary for Planning and Evaluation, US Department of Health and Human Services. November 30, 2003. Accessed December 11, 2023. https://aspe.hhs.gov/reports/state-funded-pre-kindergarten-what-evidence-shows-0

119. Whitmore Schanzenbach D, Bauer L. The Long-Term Impact of the Head Start Program. *Brookings*. August 19, 2016. Accessed December 8, 2023. https://www.brookings.edu/articles/the-long-term-impact-of-the-head-start-program/

120. Friedman-Krauss A, Barnett WS, Nores M. How Much Can High-Quality Universal Pre-K Reduce Achievement Gaps? Center for American Progress. April 5, 2016. Accessed December 8, 2023. https://www.americanprogress.org/article/how-much-can-high-quality-universal-pre-k-reduce-achievement-gaps/

References

121. How Is K–12 Education Funded? Peter G. Peterson Foundation. August 25, 2023. Accessed December 8, 2023. https://www.pgpf.org /budget-basics/how-is-k-12-education-funded

122. Jackson CK, Johnson RC, Persico C. The Effects of School Spending on Educational and Economic Outcomes: Evidence from School Finance Reforms. National Bureau of Economic Research. January 2015. https://www.doi.org/10.3386/w20847

123. Turner C, Guerra J, Zeff S, et al. Is There a Better Way to Pay for America's Schools? *National Public Radio.* May 1, 2016. Accessed December 8, 2023. https://www.npr.org/2016/05/01/476224759/is -there-a-better-way-to-pay-for-americas-schools

124. Burnette DB II. Equity in K–12 Funding More Complex Than Just Dollars. *Education Week.* June 6, 2018. Accessed December 8, 2023. https://www.edweek.org/policy-politics/equity-in-k-12-funding -more-complex-than-just-dollars/2018/06

125. School-Based Health Centers. County Health Rankings & Road-maps. February 9, 2023. Accessed December 8, 2023. https://www .countyhealthrankings.org/take-action-to-improve-health/what -works-for-health/strategies/school-based-health-centers

126. Arenson M, Hudson PJ, Lee N, Lai B. The Evidence on School-Based Health Centers: A Review. *Glob Pediatr Health.* 2019;6. https://www .doi.org/10.1177/2333794X19828745

127. Greenburg D, Dang L. Community Schools: Fostering Innovation and Transformation. *ED.gov.* June 28, 2023. Accessed December 8, 2023. https://blog.ed.gov/2023/06/community-schools-fostering -innovation-and-transformation/

128. Bloodworth MR, Horner AC. *Return on Investment of a Community School Coordinator: A Case Study.* Apex; 2019. https://www .communityschools.org/wp-content/uploads/sites/2/2020/11/ROI _Coordinator.pdf

129. Putnam RD. *Bowling Alone: The Collapse and Revival of American Community.* Touchstone ed. Simon & Schuster; 2001.

130. Wildeman C. Incarceration and Population Health in Wealthy Democracies*. *Criminology.* 2016;54(2):360–382. https://www.doi .org/10.1111/1745-9125.12107

131. Syriopoulou E, Bower H, Andersson TML, Lambert PC, Rutherford MJ. Estimating the Impact of a Cancer Diagnosis on Life Expectancy

by Socio-Economic Group for a Range of Cancer Types in England. *Br J Cancer.* 2017;117(9):1419–1426. https://www.doi.org/10.1038/bjc.2017.300

132. Davis AY. *Masked Racism: Reflections on the Prison Industrial Complex in the USA.* Lola Press; 2000;(12):52.

133. Thompson A, Tapp ST. *Criminal Victimization, 2022.* US Department of Justice, Office of Justice Programs, Bureau of Justice Statistics; 2023. https://bjs.ojp.gov/document/cv22.pdf

134. Gramlich J. What the Data Says (and Doesn't Say) About Crime in the United States. Pew Research Center. November 20, 2020. Accessed December 6, 2023. https://www.pewresearch.org/short-reads/2020/11/20/facts-about-crime-in-the-u-s/

135. Incarceration Statistics. Vera Institute of Justice. Accessed December 6, 2023. https://www.vera.org/ending-mass-incarceration/causes-of-mass-incarceration/incarceration-statistics

136. Steman D. *The Prison Paradox: More Incarceration Will Not Make Us Safer.* Vera Institute of Justice; 2017. Accessed December 6, 2023. https://www.vera.org/publications/for-the-record-prison-paradox-incarceration-not-safer

137. Harding DJ. Do Prisons Make Us Safer? *Scientific American.* June 21, 2019. Accessed December 7, 2023. https://www.scientificamerican.com/article/do-prisons-make-us-safer/

138. The Death Penalty in 2024: Executions. Death Penalty Information Center. Accessed February 25. 2025. https://deathpenaltyinfo.org/research/analysis/reports/year-end-reports/the-death-penalty-in-2024/executions

139. Nellis A. Still Life: America's Increasing Use of Life and Long-Term Sentences. *The Sentencing Project.* 2017. Accessed February 25, 2025. https://www.sentencingproject.org/app/uploads/2022/10/Still-Life.pdf

140. Lee RD, Fang X, Luo F. The Impact of Parental Incarceration on the Physical and Mental Health of Young Adults. *Pediatrics.* 2013;131(4):e1188–1195. https://www.doi.org/10.1542/peds.2012-0627

141. Hatzenbuehler ML, Keyes K, Hamilton A, Uddin M, Galea S. The Collateral Damage of Mass Incarceration: Risk of Psychiatric Morbid-

ity Among Nonincarcerated Residents of High-Incarceration Neigh-borhoods. *Am J Public Health*. 2015;105(1):138–143. https://www.doi.org/10.2105/AJPH.2014.302184

142. Moran TK. and Cooper JL. *Discretion and the Criminal Justice Process*. Associated Faculty Press; 1983.

143. Saunders J, Midgette G. A Test for Implicit Bias in Discretionary Criminal Justice Decisions. *Law and Human Behavior*. 2023;47(1):217.

144. Essex A, Hartman M. Racial and Ethnic Disparities in the Criminal Justice System. National Conference of State Legislatures; 2022. Accessed February 25, 2025. https://documents.ncsl.org/wwwncsl/Criminal-Justice/Racial-and-Ethnic-Disparities-in-the-Justice-System_v03.pdf

145. Eisinger J. Why Only One Top Banker Went to Jail for the Financial Crisis. *New York Times*. April 30, 2014. Accessed December 7, 2023. https://www.nytimes.com/2014/05/04/magazine/only-one-top-banker-jail-financial-crisis.html

146. Waller A. Man Sentenced to Life Over Theft of Hedge Clippers Is Granted Parole. *New York Times*. October 17, 2020. Accessed December 7, 2023. https://www.nytimes.com/2020/10/17/us/louisiana-habitual-offender-parole.html

147. Kim K, Becker-Cohen M, Serakos M. The Processing and Treatment of Mentally Ill Persons in the Criminal Justice System. Urban Institute. April 7, 2015. Accessed December 7, 2023. https://www.urban.org/research/publication/processing-and-treatment-mentally-ill-persons-criminal-justice-system

148. Department of Justice. Annual Determination of Average Cost of Incarceration Fee (COIF). *Federal Register*. September 22, 2023:65405–65405.

149. US Census Bureau. Real Median Personal Income in the United States. September 12, 2023. Accessed August 23, 2024. https://fred.stlouisfed.org/series/MEPAINUSA672N

150. McLaughlin M, Pettus-Davis C, Brown D, Veeh C, Renn T. *The Economic Burden of Incarceration in the United States*. Institute for Justice Research and Development. July 1, 2016. https://ijrd.csw.fsu.edu/sites/g/files/upcbnu1766/files/media/images/publication_pdfs/Economic_Burden_of_Incarceration_IJRD072016_0_0.pdf

151. EPA's Budget and Spending. United States Environmental Protection Agency. Accessed December 7, 2023. https://www.epa.gov /planandbudget/budget

152. WIC Program. Accessed December 7, 2023. https://www.ers.usda .gov/topics/food-nutrition-assistance/wic-program/

153. Sawyer W, Wagner P. Mass Incarceration: The Whole Pie 2022. Prison Policy Initiative. March 14, 2022. Accessed December 7, 2023. https://www.prisonpolicy.org/reports/pie2023.html

154. Sherman LW, Strang H. *Restorative Justice: The Evidence*. Smith Institute; 2007.

155. RJ Diversion. Full Circle Restorative Justice. Accessed December 7, 2023. https://fullcirclerj.org/programs/rj-diversion/

156. Widra E, Herring T. States of Incarceration: The Global Context 2021. Prison Policy Initiative. September 2021. Accessed December 7, 2023. https://www.prisonpolicy.org/global/2021.html

157. Taylor A. The Netherlands Has a Strange Problem: Empty Prisons. *Washington Post*. July 8, 2016. Accessed December 7, 2023. https://www.washingtonpost.com/news/worldviews/wp /2016/07/08/the-netherlands-have-a-strange-problem-empty -prisons/

158. Mauer M, Ghandnoosh N. Fewer Prisoners, Less Crime: A Tale of Three States. The Sentencing Project. Accessed January 18, 2025. https://www.sentencingproject.org/app/uploads/2022/08/Fewer -Prisoners-Less-Crime-A-Tale-of-Three-States.pdf

159. Sherman LW, Strang H, Mayo-Wilson E, Woods DJ, Ariel B. Are Restorative Justice Conferences Effective in Reducing Repeat Offending? Findings from a Campbell Systematic Review. *J Quant Criminol*. 2015;31(1):1–24. https://www.doi.org/10.1007/s10940 -014-9222-9

160. Adamczyk A. Best Places to Live for Families. *Fortune Well*. Accessed August 9, 2023. https://fortune.com/well/ranking/best-places -families/2022/ann-arbor/

161. Ann Arbor, MI is the #2 Best City to Live in the USA. *Livability*. Accessed December 7, 2023. https://livability.com/best-places /2022-top-100-best-places-to-live-in-the-us/top-100-2022-ann -arbor-mi/

162. 2023 Best Cities to Raise a Family. *Niche*. Accessed December 7, 2023. https://www.niche.com/places-to-live/search/best-cities-for -families/

163. Lewis C, Rosenfeld B. Six Years After Police Killed Aura Rosser, Community Members Say They Won't Forget Her. *Michigan Daily*. November 9, 2020. Accessed December 7, 2023. http://www .michigandaily.com/news/ann-arbor/aura-rosser-vigil/

164. Abbey-Lambertz K. No Charges for Officer Who Killed Mentally Ill Woman Who "Confronted" Police with a Knife. *HuffPost*. February 3, 2015. Accessed December 7, 2023. https://www.huffpost.com/entry /aura-rosser-killed-dave-ried-ann-arbor_n_6604458

165. Sinyangwe S, Hammond M, Hall J, et al. 2023 Police Violence Report. Mapping Police Violence. 2025. Accessed February 25, 2025. https://policeviolencereport.org/2024

166. Hill E, Tiefenthäler A, Triebert C, Jordan D, Willis H, Stein R. How George Floyd Was Killed in Police Custody. *New York Times*. June 1, 2020. Accessed December 7, 2023. https://www.nytimes.com/2020 /05/31/us/george-floyd-investigation.html

167. Oppel RA Jr, Taylor DB, Bogel-Burroughs N. What to Know About Breonna Taylor's Death. *New York Times*. November 16, 2023. Accessed December 7, 2023. https://www.nytimes.com/article /breonna-taylor-police.html

168. Feldman JM, Chen JT, Waterman PD, Krieger N. Temporal Trends and Racial/Ethnic Inequalities for Legal Intervention Injuries Treated in Emergency Departments: US Men and Women Age 15–34, 2001–2014. *J Urban Health*. 2016;93(5):797–807. https:// www.doi.org/10.1007/s11524-016-0076-3

169. Edwards F, Lee H, Esposito M. Risk of Being Killed by Police Use of Force in the United States by Age, Race–Ethnicity, and Sex. *Proc Natl Acad Sci USA*. 2019;116(34):16793–16798. https://www.doi.org /10.1073/pnas.1821204116

170. Stinson PM, Liederbach J, Lab SP, Brewer SL. *Police Integrity Lost: A Study of Law Enforcement Officers Arrested*. US Department of Justice; 2016. https://www.ojp.gov/pdffiles1/nij/grants /249850.pdf

171. Geller A, Fagan J, Tyler T, Link BG. Aggressive Policing and the Mental Health of Young Urban Men. *Am J Public Health*. 2014;

104(12):2321–2327. https://www.doi.org/10.2105/AJPH.2014
.302046

172. Gottlieb A, Wilson R. The Effect of Direct and Vicarious Police
Contact on the Educational Achievement of Urban Teens. *Children
and Youth Serv Rev.* 2019;103:190–199. https://www.doi.org/10.1016
/j.childyouth.2019.06.009

173. Legewie J, Fagan J. Aggressive Policing and the Educational
Performance of Minority Youth. *Am Sociol Rev.* 2019;84(2):220–247.
https://www.doi.org/10.1177/0003122419826020

174. Alang S, McAlpine DD, Hardeman R. Police Brutality and Mistrust in
Medical Institutions. *J Racial and Ethnic Health Disparities.* 2020;
7(4):760–768. https://www.doi.org/10.1007/s40615-020-00706-w

175. Brayne S. Surveillance and System Avoidance: Criminal Justice
Contact and Institutional Attachment. *Am Sociol Rev.* 2014;
79(3):367–391. https://www.doi.org/10.1177/0003122414530398

176. McFarland MJ, Taylor J, McFarland CAS, Friedman KL. Perceived
Unfair Treatment by Police, Race, and Telomere Length: A Nashville
Community-Based Sample of Black and White Men. *J Health
Soc Behav.* 2018;59(4):585–600. https://www.doi.org/10.1177
/0022146518811144

177. Bor J, Venkataramani AS, Williams DR, Tsai AC. Police Killings and
Their Spillover Effects on the Mental Health of Black Americans:
A Population-Based, Quasi-Experimental Study. *Lancet.* 2018;
392(10144):302–310. https://www.doi.og/10.1016/S0140-6736(18)
31130-9

178. Sewell AA. Policing the Block: Pandemics, Systemic Racism, and the
Blood of America. *City & Community.* 2020;19(3):496–505.
https://www.doi.org/10.1111/cico.12517

179. Fleming PJ, Lopez WD, Mesa H, et al. A Qualitative Study on the
Impact of the 2016 US Election on the Health of Immigrant Families
in Southeast Michigan. *BMC Public Health.* 2019;19(1):947. https://
www.doi.org/10.1186/s12889-019-7290-3

180. Lopez WD. *Separated: Family and Community in the Aftermath of
an Immigration Raid.* Johns Hopkins University Press; 2019.

181. Charbonneau A, Glaser J. Suspicion and Discretion in Policing:
How Laws and Policies Contribute to Inequity. *UC Irvine L. Rev.*
2020;11:1327.

182. Flynn S. NYPD Blasted for Bragging Post About Arrests of People for Stealing Diapers. *The Independent*. February 17, 2022. Accessed December 7, 2023. https://www.the-independent.com/news/world /americas/crime/nypd-twitter-seizure-diapers-medicine-b2017663 .html

183. Akinnibi F, Holder S, Cannon C. Cities Say They Want to Defund the Police. Their Budgets Say Otherwise. *Bloomberg*. January 12, 2021. Accessed December 7, 2023. https://www.bloomberg.com/graphics /2021-city-budget-police-funding/

184. What Policing Costs: A Look at Spending in America's Biggest Cities. Vera Institute of Justice. Accessed December 7, 2023. https://www .vera.org/publications/what-policing-costs-in-americas-biggest -cities

185. *The Challenge of Crime in a Free Society: A Report by the President's Commission on Law Enforcement and Administration of Justice*. US Government Printing Office; 1967:6. https://www.ojp.gov/sites/g /files/xyckuh241/files/archives/ncjrs/42.pdf

186. Hinton EK. *From the War on Poverty to the War on Crime: The Making of Mass Incarceration in America*. Harvard University Press; 2016.

187. Rosalsky G. When You Add More Police to a City, What Happens? *National Public Radio*. April 20, 2021. Accessed December 7, 2023. https://www.npr.org/sections/money/2021 /04/20/988769793/when-you-add-more-police-to-a-city-what -happens

188. South EC. To Combat Gun Violence, Clean Up the Neighborhood. *New York Times*. October 8, 2021. Accessed December 7, 2023. https://www.nytimes.com/2021/10/08/opinion/gun-violence-biden -philadelphia.html

189. Zimmerman MA. Want to Fight Crime? Plant Some Flowers with Your Neighbor. *The Conversation*. March 22, 2018. Accessed December 7, 2023. http://theconversation.com/want-to-fight-crime -plant-some-flowers-with-your-neighbor-91804

190. Naimi TS, Xuan Z, Coleman SM, et al. Alcohol Policies and Alcohol-Involved Homicide Victimization in the United States. *J Stud Alcohol Drugs*. 2017;78(5):781–788. https://www.doi.org/10.15288 /jsad.2017.78.781

191. Lepore J. The Invention of the Police. *The New Yorker.* July 13, 2020. Accessed August 23, 2024. https://www.newyorker.com/magazine /2020/07/20/the-invention-of-the-police

192. nicole luna. But Actually Imagine Transformative Alternatives to Policing. *Medium.* June 14, 2020. Accessed December 7, 2023. https://medium.com/@amber.hughson/but-actually-imagine -transformative-alternatives-to-policing-69a3d9afbe7e

193. The Washington Post. Dallas Police Chief: "We're Asking Cops to Do Too Much." *Denver Post.* July 12, 2016. Accessed December 7, 2023. https://www.denverpost.com/2016/07/12/dallas-police-chief-were -asking-cops-to-do-too-much/

194. Spolum MM, Lopez WD, Watkins DC, Fleming PJ. Police Violence: Reducing the Harms of Policing Through Public Health-Informed Alternative Response Programs. *Am J Public Health.* 2023;113(S1): S37-S42. https://www.doi.org/10.2105/AJPH.2022.307107

195. Watson AC, Compton MT. What Research on Crisis Intervention Teams Tells Us and What We Need to Ask. *Journal of the American Academy of Psychiatry and the Law Online.* 2019 Nov 1.

196. Episode 66: Ryan Henyard and Paul Fleming on the Coalition for Reenvisioning Our Safety. *Ann Arbor AF* podcast. Accessed December 7, 2023. https://annarboraf.com/episode-66-ryan-henyard-and -paul-fleming-on-the-coalition-for-reenvisioning-our-safety/

197. Kim ME, Chung M, Hassan S, Ritchie AJ. *Defund the Police—Invest in Community Care: A Guide to Alternative Mental Health Responses.* Interrupting Criminalization; 2021. Accessed December 7, 2023. https://www.interruptingcriminalization.com/non-police -crisis-response-guide

198. Eugene Police Crime Analysis Unit. *CAHOOTS Program Analysis.* Accessed January 18, 2025. https://www.eugene-or.gov/Document Center/View/56717/CAHOOTS-Program-Analysis

199. What Is CAHOOTS? White Bird Clinic. October 29, 2020. Accessed December 8, 2023. https://whitebirdclinic.org/what-is -cahoots/

200. Dee TS, Pyne J. A Community Response Approach to Mental Health and Substance Abuse Crises Reduced Crime. *Sci Adv.* 2022;8(23): eabm2106. https://www.doi.org/10.1126/sciadv.abm2106

201. Jackson RJ, Minjares R, Naumoff KS, Shrimali BP, Martin LK. Agriculture Policy Is Health Policy. *J Hunger Environ Nutr.* 2009; 4(3–4):393–408. https://www.doi.org/10.1080/19320240903321367

202. Fleming PJ, Novak NL, Lopez WD. US Immigration Law Enforcement Practices and Health Inequities. *Am J Prev Med.* 2019;57(6):858–861. https://www.doi.org/10.1016/j.amepre.2019.07.019

203. Leigh JP, Chakalov B. Labor Unions and Health: A Literature Review of Pathways and Outcomes in the Workplace. *Prev Med Rep.* 2021;24:101502. https://www.doi.org/10.1016/j.pmedr.2021 .101502

204. Bilick S, Akemi Piatt A. Tax Day: What's Health Equity Got to Do with It? *Medium.* April 15, 2021. Accessed December 9, 2023. https://humanimpact-hip.medium.com/tax-day-whats-health -equity-got-to-do-with-it-ba4b3a0a9629

205. Litman T. Transportation and Public Health. *Ann Rev Public Health.* 2013;34(1):217–233. https://www.doi.org/10.1146/annurev-publhealth -031912-114502

206. Executive Order 13958, Establishing the President's Advisory 1776 Commission, November 2, 2020.

207. Alleyne A. Book Banning, Curriculum Restrictions, and the Politicization of US Schools. Center for American Progress; 2022. https:// www.americanprogress.org/article/book-banning-curriculum -restrictions-and-the-politicization-of-us-schools.

208. Hannah-Jones N. From the Magazine: "It Is Time for Reparations." *New York Times.* June 24, 2020. Accessed October 18, 2024. https://www.nytimes.com/interactive/2020/06/24/magazine /reparations-slavery.html.

209. Angier N. Do Races Differ? Not Really, Genes Show. *New York Times.* August 22, 2000. Accessed December 11, 2023. https://www .nytimes.com/2000/08/22/science/do-races-differ-not-really-genes -show.html.

210. Ignatiev N. *How the Irish Became White.* Routledge; 2009.

211. Davenport L. The Fluidity of Racial Classifications. *Annu Rev Polit Sci.* 2019;23(23):221–240. https://www.doi.org/10.1146/annurev -polisci-060418-042801

212. Lewis C, Cohen PR, Bahl D, Levine EM, Khaliq W. Race and Ethnic Categories: A Brief Review of Global Terms and Nomenclature. *Cureus.* 2023;15(7):e41253. https://www.doi.org/10.7759/cureus.41253

213. Kendi IX. *Stamped from the Beginning: The Definitive History of Racist Ideas in America.* 1st trade paperback ed. Bold Type Books; 2017.

214. Painter NI. *The History of White People.* 1st paperback ed. Norton; 2011.

215. Wolfe B. Indentured Servants in Colonial Virginia. Encyclopedia Virginia. December 7, 2020. Accessed October 18, 2024. https://encyclopediavirginia.org/entries/indentured-servants-in-colonial-virginia/

216. General Court Responds to Runaway Servants and Slaves (1640). Encyclopedia Virgina. Accessed February 25, 2025. https://encyclopediavirginia.org/primary-documents/general-court-responds-to-runaway-servants-and-slaves-1640/.

217. General Assembly. "An act to repeale a former law makeing Indians and others ffree" (1682). *Encyclopedia Virginia.* December 7, 2020. https://encyclopediavirginia.org/entries/an-act-to-repeale-a-former-law-makeing-indians-and-others-ffree-1682/

218. General Assembly. "An act for suppressing outlying slaves" (1691). *Encyclopedia Virginia.* December 7, 2020. Accessed December 12, 2023. https://encyclopediavirginia.org/entries/an-act-for-suppressing-outlying-slaves-1691/

219. Cox A. Settler Colonialism. *Oxford Bibliographies.* July 26, 2017. https://www.oxfordbibliographies.com/display/document/obo-9780190221911/obo-9780190221911-0029.xml

220. Magazine S, Lidz F. Following in the Footsteps of Balboa. *Smithsonian Magazine.* September 2013. Accessed December 12, 2023. https://www.smithsonianmag.com/history/following-in-the-footsteps-of-balboa-803409/

221. Heidler DS, Heidler JT. Manifest Destiny. *Britannica.* October 17, 2023. https://www.britannica.com/event/Manifest-Destiny

222. Immigration and Relocation in US History. Library of Congress. Accessed October 18, 2024. https://www.loc.gov/classroom-materials/immigration/native-american/

223. Vazquez J. Forced Removal of Native Americans. Equal Justice Initiative. July 1, 2016. Accessed October 18, 2024. https://eji.org/news/history-racial-injustice-forced-removal -native-americans/

224. Allen DW, Leonard B. Late Homesteading: Native Land Dispossession Through Strategic Occupation. *Am Polit Sci Rev*. February 16, 2024:1–15. https://www.doi.org/10.1017/S000305542 3001466

225. Indian Treaties and the Removal Act of 1830. United States Department of State. Accessed October 18, 2024. https://history.state.gov /milestones/1830-1860/indian-treaties

226. Watson BA. *Buying America from the Indians: Johnson v. McIntosh and the History of Native Land Rights*. University of Oklahoma Press; 2012.

227. President Andrew Jackson's Message to Congress "On Indian Removal" (1830). National Archives. May 10, 2022. https://www .archives.gov/milestone-documents/jacksons-message-to-congress -on-indian-removal

228. Trail of Tears: Definition, Date & Cherokee Nation. HISTORY. September 26, 2023. Accessed December 9, 2023. https://www .history.com/topics/native-american-history/trail-of-tears

229. Thornton R. Cherokee Population Losses During the Trail of Tears: A New Perspective and a New Estimate. *Ethnohistory*. 1984;31(4): 289–300. https://www.doi.org/10.2307/482714

230. Invasion of America. ArcGIS. Accessed December 9, 2023. https:// usg.maps.arcgis.com/apps/webappviewer/index.html?id=eb6ca76 e008543a89349ff2517db47e6

231. Nov. 1, 1879 | Federal Government Separates Native Children from Families in Efforts at Forced Assimilation. A History of Racial Injustice. https://calendar.eji.org/racial-injustice/nov/01

232. American Indian Boarding Schools Haunt Many. *National Public Radio*. May 12, 2008. https://www.npr.org/2008/05/12/16516865 /american-indian-boarding-schools-haunt-many

233. Wolfe P. Settler Colonialism and the Elimination of the Native. *J Genocide Res*. 2006;8(4):387–409. https://www.doi.org/10.1080 /14623520601056240

234. United Nations. Convention on the Prevention and Punishment of the Crime of Genocide. December 9, 1948. https://www.un.org/en /genocideprevention/documents/publications-and-resources /Genocide_Convention_75thAnniversary_2023.pdf

235. Brave Heart MY, DeBruyn LM. The American Indian Holocaust: Healing Historical Unresolved Grief. *Am Indian Alsk Nativ Ment Health Res (1987)*. 1998;8(2):56–78.

236. Gone JP, Hartmann WE, Pomerville A, Wendt DC, Klem SH, Burrage RL. The Impact of Historical Trauma on Health Outcomes for Indigenous Populations in the USA and Canada: A Systematic Review. *Am Psychol*. 2019;74(1):20–35. https://www.doi.org/10.1037 /amp0000338

237. US Constitution. ArtI.S8.C4.1.2.3 Early US Naturalization Laws. *Constitution Annotated*. https://constitution.congress.gov/browse /essay/artI-S8-C4-1-2-3/ALDE_00013163/

238. Landmark Legislation: The Fourteenth Amendment. United States Senate. https://www.senate.gov/about/origins-foundations/senate -and-constitution/14th-amendment.htm

239. Smith ML. Race, Nationality, and Reality. *National Archives*. 2022. https://www.archives.gov/publications/prologue/2002/summer /immigration-law-1

240. Biewen J, Kumanyika C. S2 E10: Citizen Thind. Scene on Radio podcast. June 14, 2017. Accessed December 12, 2023. https:// sceneonradio.org/episode-40-citizen-thind-seeing-white-part-10/

241. Biewen J, Kumanyika C. S2 E10: Citizen Thind. *Scene on Radio* podcast. June 14, 2017. Accessed December 12, 2023. https:// sceneonradio.org/episode-40-citizen-thind-seeing-white-part-10/

242. Bauer M, Stewart M. Close to Slavery: Guestworker Programs in the United States. Southern Poverty Law Center. February 19, 2013. https://www.splcenter.org/20130218/close-slavery-guestworker -programs-united-states

243. Molina N. Borders, Laborers, and Racialized Medicalization Mexican Immigration and US Public Health Practices in the 20th Century. *Am J Public Health*. 2011;101(6):1024–1031. https:// www.doi.org/10.2105/AJPH.2010.300056

244. Handal AJ, Iglesias-Ríos L. Michigan's Thousands of Farmworkers Are Unprotected, Poorly Paid, Uncounted and Often Exploited.

The Conversation. July 15, 2024. Accessed October 18, 2024. https://theconversation.com/michigans-thousands-of-farmworkers-are-unprotected-poorly-paid-uncounted-and-often-exploited-231152

245. Hartocollis A. How the Term "Affirmative Action" Came to Be. *New York Times*. October 31, 2022. https://www.nytimes.com/2022/10/31/us/politics/affirmative-action-history.html

246. Katznelson I. *When Affirmative Action Was White: An Untold History of Racial Inequality in Twentieth-Century America*. 1st paperback ed. W. W. Norton; 2006.

247. Schneider GL. The G.I. Bill. Bill of Rights Institute. Accessed October 18, 2024. https://billofrightsinstitute.org/essays/the-gi-bill/

248. Biewen J, Kumanyika C, Hayes-Greene D. S2 E13: White Affirmative Action. *Scene on Radio* podcast. August 9, 2017. Accessed December 12, 2023. https://sceneonradio.org/episode-44-white-affirmative-action-seeing-white-part-13/

249. Rothstein R. *The Color of Law: A Forgotten History of How Our Government Segregated America*. Liveright Publishing, a division of W. W. Norton; 2018.

250. Gross T. A "Forgotten History" of How the US Government Segregated America. *Fresh Air*. National Public Radio. May 3, 2017. Accessed October 18, 2024. https://www.npr.org/2017/05/03/526655831/a-forgotten-history-of-how-the-u-s-government-segregated-america

251. Ray R, Perry AM, Harshbarger D, Elizondo S, Gibbons A. Homeownership, Racial Segregation, and Policy Solutions to Racial Wealth Equity. *Brookings*. September 1, 2021. Accessed October 18, 2024. https://www.brookings.edu/articles/homeownership-racial-segregation-and-policies-for-racial-wealth-equity/

252. Swope CB, Hernández D, Cushing LJ. The Relationship of Historical Redlining with Present-Day Neighborhood Environmental and Health Outcomes: A Scoping Review and Conceptual Model. *J Urban Health*. 2022;99(6):959–983. https://www.doi.org/10.1007/s11524-022-00665-z

253. Huang SJ, Sehgal NJ. Association of Historic Redlining and Present-Day Health in Baltimore. *PLOS ONE*. 2022;17(1):e0261028. https://www.doi.org/10.1371/journal.pone.0261028

254. Barber C. Public Enemy Number One: A Pragmatic Approach to America's Drug Problem. Richard Nixon Foundation. June 29, 2016. Accessed December 11, 2023. https://www.nixonfoundation.org /2016/06/26404/

255. GAO. Drug Control: Office of National Drug Control Policy Met Some Strategy Requirements but Needs a Performance Evaluation Plan. US Government Accountability Office. December 19, 2022. https://www.gao.gov/products/gao-23-105508

256. Baum D. Legalize It All: How to Win the War on Drugs. *Harper's Magazine.* April 2016. Accessed December 11, 2023. https://harpers .org/archive/2016/04/legalize-it-all/

257. Hudak J. Biden Should End America's Longest War: The War on Drugs. *Brookings.* September 24, 2021. https://www.brookings.edu /articles/biden-should-end-americas-longest-war-the-war-on-drugs/

258. Alexander M. *The New Jim Crow: Mass Incarceration in the Age of Colorblindness.* Rev. ed. New Press; 2012.

259. Cracks in the System: 20 Years of the Unjust Federal Crack Cocaine Law. American Civil Liberties Union. October 26, 2006. https:// www.aclu.org/documents/cracks-system-20-years-unjust-federal -crack-cocaine-law

260. Lopez G. Black and White Americans Use Drugs at Similar Rates. One Group Is Punished More for It. *Vox.* March 17, 2015. https:// www.vox.com/2015/3/17/8227569/war-on-drugs-racism

261. OHCHR. UN Experts Call for End to Global "War on Drugs." United Nations Office of the High Commissioner for Human Rights. June 23, 2023. https://www.ohchr.org/en/press-releases/2023/06 /un-experts-call-end-global-war-drugs

262. Thrush G. Justice Dept. Revises Rules for Drug Cases to Address Racial Disparities. *New York Times.* December 16, 2022. https://www .nytimes.com/2022/12/16/us/politics/justice-dept-crack-cocaine.html

263. Nellis A, Komar L. The First Step Act: Ending Mass Incarceration in Federal Prisons. The Sentencing Project. August 22, 2023. Accessed December 11, 2023. https://www.sentencingproject.org/policy-brief /the-first-step-act-ending-mass-incarceration-in-federal-prisons/

264. Sclerotic. *Oxford English Dictionary.* Oxford University Press. Accessed January 18, 2025. https://languages.oup.com/

265. Green EL, Montague Z. Trump Signs Two Orders to Dismantle Equity Policies. *New York Times.* January 20, 2025. https://www.nytimes.com/2025/01/20/us/politics/trump-transgender-race-education.html

266. Brand Story. Civilla. Accessed October 24, 2024. https://civilla.org/brand-story

267. 2016 Michigan House of Representatives Election. *Wikipedia*; 2023. https://en.wikipedia.org/w/index.php?title=2016_Michigan_House_of_Representatives_election

268. 2012 Michigan House of Representatives Election. *Wikipedia.*; 2023. Accessed December 11, 2023. https://en.wikipedia.org/w/index.php?title=2012_Michigan_House_of_Representatives_election

269. Beggin R. One Woman's Facebook Post Leads to Michigan Vote Against Gerrymandering. *Bridge Michigan.* November 7, 2018. https://www.bridgemi.com/michigan-government/one-womans-facebook-post-leads-michigan-vote-against-gerrymandering

270. 2022 Michigan Official General Election Results. *Michigan.gov.* November 8, 2022. https://mielections.us/election/results/2022GEN_CENR.html

271. Benjamin R. *Viral Justice: How We Grow the World We Want.* Princeton University Press; 2022.

272. Kishimoto K. Anti-Racist Pedagogy: From Faculty's Self-Reflection to Organizing Within and Beyond the Classroom. *Race Ethnicity and Education.* 2016;21(4):540–554. https://www.doi.org/10.1080/13613324.2016.1248824

273. Costello M. Art for Community. Molly Costello Art & Design. Accessed January 18, 2025. https://www.mollycostello.com/art-community

274. Jennings WG, Piquero AR, Reingle JM. On the Overlap Between Victimization and Offending: A Review of the Literature. *Aggression and Violent Behavior.* 2012;17(1):16–26. https://www.doi.org/10.1016/j.avb.2011.09.003

275. Tran Myhre K "Guante." *A Love Song, A Death Rattle, A Battle Cry.* 2nd ed. Button Poetry/Exploding Pinecone Press; 2017.

276. Malcolm X, Haley A. *The Autobiography of Malcolm X.* 1st ed. [Nachdr.]. Ballantine Books; 1999.

277. Freire P. *Pedagogy of the Oppressed*. Penguin Classics; 2017.

278. Sirolli E. *Want to Help Someone? Shut Up and Listen!* TEDx-EQChCh; September 2012. https://www.ted.com/talks/ernesto _sirolli_want_to_help_someone_shut_up_and_listen/transcript

279. @prisonculture. Questions I regularly ask myself when I'm outraged by justice: 1. What resources exist so I can better educate myself? 2. Who's already doing work around this injustice? 3. Do I have the capacity to offer concrete support & help to them? 4. How can I be constructive. (Posted on X; since deleted).

280. Broadfoot M. We Need to Ground Truth Assumptions about Gene Therapy. *Scientific American*. November 1, 2021. Accessed October 24, 2024. https://www.scientificamerican.com/article/we-need -to-ground-truth-assumptions-about-gene-therapy/

281. Creary MS. Bounded Justice and the Limits of Health Equity. *J Law Med Ethics*. 2021;49(2):241–256. https://www.doi.org/10.1017/jme .2021.34

282. Affirmatively Furthering Fair Housing. US Department of Housing and Urban Development. https://www.hud.gov/AFFH.

283. Hannah-Jones N. *Living Apart: How the Government Betrayed a Landmark Civil Rights Law*. ProPublica; 2012.

284. Miller C, Stassun K. A Test That Fails. *Nature*. 2014;510:303–304.

285. Clayton V. The Problem with the GRE. *The Atlantic*. March 1, 2016. https://www.theatlantic.com/education/archive/2016/03/the -problem-with-the-gre/471633/

286. Miller CW, Zwickl BM, Posselt JR, Silvestrini RT, Hodapp T. Typical Physics Ph.D. Admissions Criteria Limit Access to Underrepresented Groups but Fail to Predict Doctoral Completion. *Sci Adv*. 2019;5(1): eaat7550. https://www.doi.org/10.1126/sciadv.aat7550

287. Hall JD, O'Connell AB, Cook JG. Predictors of Student Productivity in Biomedical Graduate School Applications. *PLOS ONE*. 2017; 12(1):e0169121. https://www.doi.org/10.1371/journal.pone.0169121

288. Policy Briefs. American Public Health Association. Accessed January 18, 2025. https://www.apha.org/Policies-and-Advocacy /Public-Health-Policy-Statements

289. Netburn D. The Concerted Campaign That Got Public Health Experts to Declare Racist Policing a Crisis. *Los Angeles Times*.

October 20, 2020. https://www.latimes.com/science/story/2020-10
-20/how-police-violence-became-a-public-health-issue

290. Arango T, Dewan S. More Than Half of Police Killings Are Misla-
beled, New Study Says. *New York Times.* September 30, 2021.
Accessed December 11, 2023. https://www.nytimes.com/2021/09
/30/us/police-killings-undercounted-study.html

291. Ganz M. Organizing: People, Power and Change. In *The Commons.*
Leading Change Network and the New Organizing Institute; 2014:
16–20. Accessed October 24, 2024. https://commonslibrary.org
/organizing-people-power-and-change-the-one-on-one-meeting/

292. DeSimone DC. Why Are Some Groups of People More at Risk of
Being Affected by COVID-19? Mayo Clinic. Accessed October 24,
2024. https://www.mayoclinic.org/diseases-conditions/coronavirus
/expert-answers/coronavirus-infection-by-race/faq-20488802

293. IISC. Illustrating Equality VS Equity. Interaction Institute for Social
Change. January 14, 2016. https://interactioninstitute.org/illustrating
-equality-vs-equity/

294. Jarow O. Basic Income Is Less Radical than You Think. *Vox.*
October 13, 2023. Accessed October 24, 2024. https://www.vox.com
/future-perfect/2023/10/13/23914745/basic-income-radical
-economy-poverty-capitalism-taxes

295. What Is Basic Income? Stanford Basic Income Lab. Accessed October 24, 2024. https://basicincome.stanford.edu/about/what-is-ubi/

296. The Child Tax Credit: What You Need to Know. University of
Michigan. Accessed October 24, 2024. https://poverty.umich.edu
/child-tax-credit/

297. Tatum BD. *Why Are All the Black Kids Sitting Together in the
Cafeteria? And Other Conversations About Race.* 3rd trade paperback ed. Basic Books; 2017.

298. Jones CP. Toward the Science and Practice of Anti-Racism: Launching a National Campaign Against Racism. *Ethn Dis.* 2018;28(Suppl
1):231–234. https://pmc.ncbi.nlm.nih.gov/articles/PMC6092166/

299. Fleming PJ, Stone LC, Creary MS, et al. Antiracism and Community-
Based Participatory Research: Synergies, Challenges, and Opportunities. *Am J Public Health.* 2023;113(1):70–78. https://www.doi.org
/10.2105/AJPH.2022.307114

300. Ford CL, Airhihenbuwa CO. The Public Health Critical Race Methodology: Praxis for Antiracism Research. *Soc Sci Med.* 2010;71(8):1390–1398. https://www.doi.org/10.1016/j.socscimed.2010.07.030

301. Crenshaw K. Mapping the Margins: Intersectionality, Identity Politics, and Violence against Women of Color. *Stanford Law Review.* 1991;43(6):1241–1299. https://www.doi.org/10.2307/1229039

302. Combahee River Collective. The Combahee River Collective Statement. April 1977. Accessed February 25, 2025. http://circuitous.org/scraps/combahee.html

303. Collins PH. *Black Feminist Thought: Knowledge, Consciousness, and the Politics of Empowerment.* Hyman; 1990.

304. Moraga C, Anzaldúa G, eds. *This Bridge Called My Back: Writings by Radical Women of Color.* Persephone Press; 1981.

305. *Promotion of National Unity and Reconciliation.* Act 34.; 1995. https://www.justice.gov.za/legislation/acts/1995-034.pdf.

306. Ibhawoh B. Do Truth and Reconciliation Commissions Heal Divided Nations? *The Conversation.* January 23, 2019. Accessed September 7, 2023. https://theconversation.com/do-truth-and-reconciliation-commissions-heal-divided-nations-109925

307. Truth, Racial Healing, and Transformation. W. K. Kellogg Foundation. Accessed January 18, 2025. https://healourcommunities.org/

308. Lee B. *H.Con.Res.19: Urging the Establishment of a United States Commission on Truth, Racial Healing, and Transformation*; 2021.

309. Williams M. Culture Shift Podcast Episode 08: Healing Racism. The Taproot of America with Dr. Gail Christopher, Former Senior Advisor and Vice President of the W. K. Kellogg Foundation. *Culture Shift Agency.* August 31, 2020. Accessed December 3, 2023. https://www.cultureshiftagency.com/blog/2020/8/28/culture-shift-podcast-08-healing-racism-the-taproot-of-america-with-dr-gail-christopher

310. Jackson Lee S. *H.R. 40: Commission to Study and Develop Reparation Proposals for African-Americans Act*; 2021. https://www.congress.gov/bill/117th-congress/house-bill/40

311. McCammon S. The Story Behind "40 Acres and a Mule." *All Things Considered.* National Public Radio. Accessed October 24, 2024. https://www.npr.org/sections/codeswitch/2015/01/12/376781165/the-story-behind-40-acres-and-a-mule

312. *126-R 19 A Resolution: Establishing a City of Evanston Funding Source Devoted to Local Reparations*; 2019. https://www.city ofevanston.org/home/showpublisheddocument/90573/638249 272128130000

313. Vigdor N. North Carolina City Approves Reparations for Black Residents. *New York Times*. July 16, 2020. Accessed December 3, 2023. https://www.nytimes.com/2020/07/16/us/reparations -asheville-nc.html

314. Darity WA, Mullen AK. *From Here to Equality: Reparations for Black Americans in the Twenty-First Century*. 2nd ed. University of North Carolina Press; 2022.

315. Rush C. Voters OK Drastic Overhaul of City Hall in Portland, Oregon. AP News. November 15, 2022. Accessed September 6, 2023. https://apnews.com/article/2022-midterm-elections -oregon-portland-homelessness-cc258eec39d938dab7dfa0e359 72d7f7

316. Beyer DS Jr. *Fair Representation Act, H.R. 3863*; 2021. https://www .congress.gov/bill/117th-congress/house-bill/3863

317. What is PB? Participatory Budgeting Project. Accessed September 6, 2023. https://www.participatorybudgeting.org/what-is-pb/

318. Community-Led Recovery. Democracy Beyond Elections. Accessed September 8, 2023. https://www.democracybeyondelections.org /wp-content/uploads/2022/12/DBE_ARPA_CaseStudy_Central Fallsvfinal.pdf

319. The People's Budget Process. The People's Budget Seattle. Accessed December 3, 2023. https://pbseattle.org/processes/peoples budget

320. "Announcing the Winning People's Budget Projects!" The People's Budget Seattle. Accessed February 27, 2025. https://pbseattle.org /processes/peoplesbudget/f/15/posts/14

321. Colin C. What If Public Funds Were Controlled by the Public? *New York Times*. April 18, 2022. Accessed November 27, 2023. https:// www.nytimes.com/2022/04/18/us/participatory-budgeting-shari -davis.html

322. Participatory Policy-Making. Democracy Beyond Elections. Accessed November 27, 2023. https://www.democracybeyondelections.org /policy/

323. Demos Helsinki. Accessed November 27, 2023. https://demoshel sinki.fi/

324. Vasconcellos B, Sigora J, Sokero M, Mertsola S, Vourdaki A. From Fortress to Foresight: A New Way of Governing Migration. Demos Helsinki. April 6, 2023. Accessed December 4, 2023. https:// demoshelsinki.fi/julkaisut/a-new-way-of-governing-migration/

325. Vasconcellos B, Sigora J, Sokero M. Anticipatory Migration Policy in North Macedonia. Demos Helsinki. April 27, 2022. Accessed November 27, 2023. https://demoshelsinki.fi/referenssit/anticipatory -migration-policy-in-north-macedonia/

326. Annala M, Leppänen J, Mertsola S. Humble Government: How to Realize Ambitious Reforms Prudently. Demos Helsinki. December 14, 2020. Accessed November 27, 2023. https://demoshelsinki.fi /julkaisut/the-more-complex-and-uncertain-a-policy-issue-is-the -more-useful-it-is-to-approach-it-through-humility/

327. Fry R, Carolina Aragão, Hurst K, Parker K. *In a Growing Share of US Marriages, Husbands and Wives Earn About the Same.* Pew Research Center; 2023. https://www.pewresearch.org/social-trends /2023/04/13/in-a-growing-share-of-u-s-marriages-husbands-and -wives-earn-about-the-same/

328. Bicchieri C. *The Grammar of Society: The Nature and Dynamics of Social Norms.* Cambridge University Press; 2006.

329. Perkins HW, Meilman PW, Leichliter JS, Cashin JR, Presley CA. Misperceptions of the Norms for the Frequency of Alcohol and Other Drug Use on College Campuses. *J Am College Health.* 1999;47(6): 253–258. https://doi.org/10.1080/07448489909595656

330. Empowering Community Leaders for Positive Change: María Militzer. University of Michigan School of Public Health. July 14, 2020. https://sph.umich.edu/stories/2020posts/maria-militzer. html

331. Mixed-Status Families Ineligible for CARES Act Federal Pandemic Stimulus Checks. Migration Policy Institute. May 2020. https:// www.migrationpolicy.org/content/mixed-status-families-ineligible -pandemic-stimulus-checks#

332. Spade D. Solidarity Not Charity. *Social Text.* 2020;38(1):136. https://www.doi.org/10.1215/01642472-7971139

333. A Huey P. Newton Story: Community Survival Programs. Public Broadcasting Service. Accessed August 23, 2024. https://www.pbs.org/hueypnewton/actions/actions_survival.html

334. Massie VM. The Most Radical Thing the Black Panthers Did Was Give Kids Free Breakfast *Vox*. October 15, 2016. Accessed October 24, 2024. https://www.vox.com/2016/2/14/10981986/black-panthers-breakfast-beyonce

335. Lukes S. *Power: A Radical View*. 3rd ed. Red Globe Press; 2021.

336. Heller JC, Little OM, Faust V, et al. Theory in Action: Public Health and Community Power Building for Health Equity. *J Public Health Manag Pract*. 2023;29(1):33–38. https://doi.org/10.1097/PHH.0000000000001681

337. Using Our Power: Power Mapping. In *Advocating for Policy Change*. Detroit Community-Academic Urban Research Center. Accessed October 24, 2024. https://legacy.detroiturc.org/policy-manual-overview.html

338. Lyons O. An Iroquois Perspective. In Vecsey C, Venables RW, eds. *American Indian Environments: Ecological Issues in Native American History*. Syracuse University Press; 1980:171–174.

Index

Index

Index

Index

Index

Index

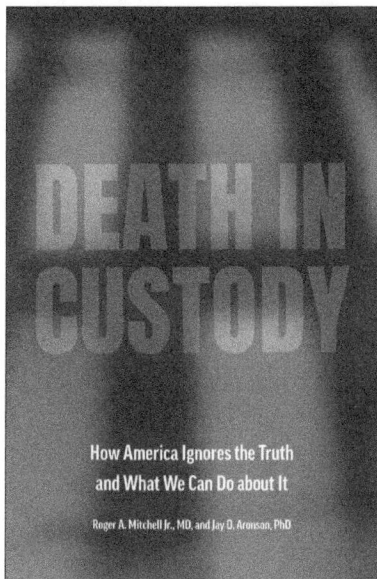

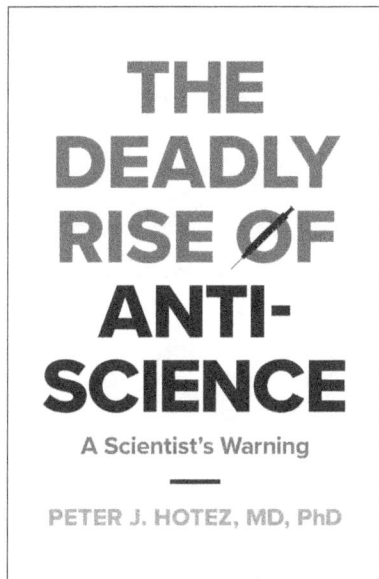

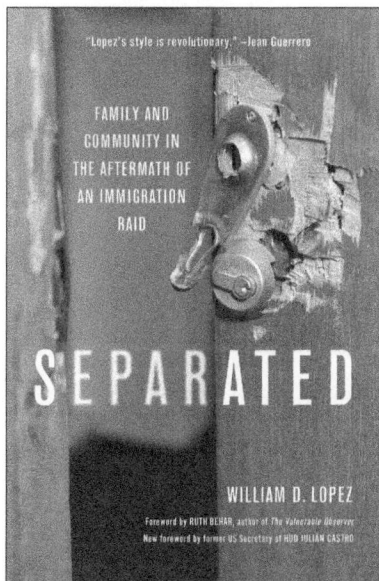

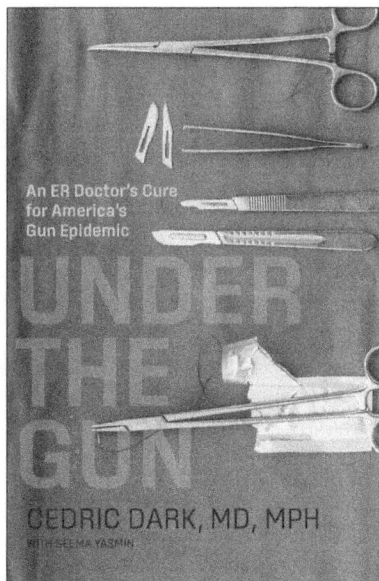